GENOCIDE!

HOW YOUR DOCTOR'S DIETARY

IGNORANCE WILL

KILL YOU !!!!

BY JAMES EDWARD CARLSON B.S., D.O., M.B.A., J.D.

ISBN: 1-4196-8582-1
ISBN-13: 9781419685828

Visit www.booksurge.com to order additional copies.

ACKNOWLEDGEMENTS

This book is dedicated to my patients who in less than six months I had told one thing and then another, much to my chagrin; but yet you still believed in me. Thank you.

I also wish to thank Sean 'The Big Kahuna' Gallagher for his tireless effort in editing my initial manuscript. I take full responsibility for any remaining errors.

Thanks also go to Thomas McIntyre for his thoughtful and insightful comments. Sorry, I just could not change the title.

Special thanks are also extended to Monica and Natalie for putting up with me during the writing of this book. I love you both. I also want to acknowledge and thank Felicia Sabatelli for reading my pregnancy chapter and offering helpful advice.

For Maggie and Jimmy

May you always know the danger of the carb, and fear not fat

and cholesterol.

My Love Always,

Dad.

OUR LIVES ARE BASED ON WHAT IS REASONABLE

AND COMMON SENSE, THE TRUTH IS APT

TO BE NEITHER

-*Zen proverb*

PREFACE

I feel compelled to write this book, not to add to the countless dietary books already on the market, but to tell the truth. To tell the truth about what has been working in my practice, over the last nine years, to help thousands of people regain control over their lives. These individuals, who suffered from a multitude of medical diseases, were helped and oftentimes cured, through simple dietary changes.

With the current information being disseminated by the popular press and well-funded three letter organizations, millions of people are being maimed and killed each year, because they believe what theses entities are endorsing. Millions of people are suffering and dying each year because they believe, based on no factual evidence, that what they are being told is true. The title GENOCIDE reflects the fact that not only are millions of people dying right here in America, but all over the world as well; all due to the continued grotesque dissemination of incorrect dietary beliefs. Unfortunately, people will continue to die and suffer horrible medical consequences and tragedies, unless the truth, a truth I know and have witnessed first hand in my clinical practice, is told.

I will clearly and logically present the truth about diet in the pages to follow. Sure some, maybe most people will state what I say is wrong. But that is their belief. The evidence I can show, the truth I can reveal, will hopefully allow millions, I wish the world, to be and stay healthy, for as long as their life on this planet.

Someone once said that it's not true because it works; it works because it's true. We will start our discussion with this premise in mind. Throughout this book, I will make statements only if I have seen it work in clinical practice. Remember, what I am about to say has worked on thousands of my patients over nine years of implementing a particular dietary plan into my patient's lives. This dietary plan worked for these patients, because it is true. Please remember this as you read this book.

I will keep the reading simple. For those of you who wish to engage in further inquiry, I will provide the references. For those physicians who hold any doubt about the information I am about to reveal, I was once you; nine years ago. Unfortunately, it will be physicians, dieticians, and nutritionists, all of who were taught incorrectly about diet, who will be my greatest critics. Even though what I write is true and can be proven through presentation of real, tangible, scientific evidence, there will still be doubt.

That is too bad. Actually, it is an absolute tragedy. Through the ignorance of the very individuals who are supposed to supply us with the knowledge on how to eat healthy, millions and millions of people continue to die each year. Yes, that does indeed constitute genocide.

Millions of people continue to die each year!

And will continue to die, unless the truth is told. And I am here to tell it.

Today. Tomorrow. Always. Remember,

IT WORKS BECAUSE IT IS TRUE.

INTRODUCTION

It is March 30, 2007 as I finally sit down to tell, hopefully the world, the correct way to eat. This book is not an exposition on the ACCEPTED way to eat, but the PROPER way to eat. It all began for me approximately 10 years ago, when I was diagnosed with high blood pressure, referred to as hypertension in medical talk. In addition, my good cholesterol known as the HDL was low. At this point in my life I was easily fifty pounds overweight, so I was not too surprised that my blood pressure was high and my HDL was low.

I decided that I should start myself on a diet and I began the accepted approach to dieting. Yes, this was the classic low fat, low cholesterol diet, gleaned from the famous Framingham Heart Study. Since I can be really strict with dieting when I want to, I began following a very low fat, low cholesterol diet plan.

Much to my surprise I gained weight, my blood pressure went higher and my HDL went even lower. But was I really surprised? I had told thousands of patients over the years to follow this particular dietary regimen; and I knew it did not work.

I knew it did not work.

This wasn't a knowledge that was obvious to me, more of like a subliminal understanding, as I had never really seen low fat, low cholesterol diets work in the past. I continued to place my patients on low fat, low cholesterol diets because that was what I was taught to do in medical school and residency.

So I continued to counsel my patients dietarily, about low fat, low cholesterol diets, throwing in that if the diet does not work, we could start medication. And I knew, most of the time, we would have to.

If the diet does not work?

If?

I am truly embarrassed to say that I never actually gave much thought as to why the vast majority of my patients did not respond to the low fat, low cholesterol diets. I implicitly knew that the diet did not work, because at the same visit I would talk about diet, I would talk about the possibility of diet failure, and the use of medications.

What was wrong with me? Why did I not stop and think about why the diet was not working? Was cholesterol elevated in my patient's blood because they were deficient in cholesterol lowering medications? Were blood pressures really elevated because my patient's blood was deficient in blood pressure lowering medications? Or blood sugars elevated because of a deficiency in one of the latest sugar lowering drugs? Why did I not smell the proverbial coffee? Why was I so *stupid*?

I really don't think I'm all that dumb. I obtained my undergraduate degree in biochemistry from Cornell, graduated from Medical School, and was Chief Resident during my Family Medicine residency. How could I have been so darn ignorant? Why did I not question what I knew and saw was not working? Why did I just reach for medications when the so-called accepted diet did not work?

Why?

Why?

Because that was the way I was trained!!!!

Let's see, it's called Medical School because you go there to learn how to use medicine. You do not go to medical school to learn how to use diet to control diseases. When I was in medical school we only received two weeks of nutritional instruction, taught by an overweight dietician.

Let me tell you something, the way one is trained in medical school stifles any chance at creativity or free thought. We are taught what to do and when to do it. We are not taught to think as a free mind in medical school. Because of this, we are indoctrinated with all the mistakes in thinking that our predecessors demonstrated before us.

Indoctrinated, wow, heavy; but true. We are not taught *how* to think, we are taught *what* to think. Because of this, when we are told in medical school, residency, and through conferences and journal readings to start low fat, low cholesterol diets; we do it without thinking.

WE DO IT WITHOUT THINKING!

Just like cattle to the slaughter, or should I say, like humans to the cath lab, or to dialysis or to chemo…we do it without thinking…

Well, wait a minute; I shouldn't just pick on the medical circle. With all due respect, we are, shall I use the word, indoctrinated again, at a very early age. We are told in elementary and high school that low fat, low cholesterol diets are correct. We learn it in college, we read it in the paper, see it on TV, and hear it on the radio. How could low fat, low cholesterol diets be wrong, when everyone knows, just knows, that this is the correct diet to be on.

So the reason I did not question the fact, (and it is very important my reader sees the word FACT for what it is) that almost everyone I placed on low fat, low cholesterol diets needed medication, was because I was trained never to question what I was told by my instructors. I was conditioned to just accept, not question, medical authority. And so I did not.

So I did not question the powers that be. It was not until I came across a wonderful book, *Protein Power*, by Mary and

Dan Eades, that my life, both professionally and personally, was changed forever.

It is important to note that my undergraduate training was in biochemistry and cellular physiology. It is also important that when I found out I had elevated blood pressure and low HDL, I started myself on a low fat, low cholesterol diet. Remember also that the diet did not work. I gained weight, my blood pressure went higher and my HDL decreased.

Guess what I did to myself next. That's right! I started myself on medications for blood pressure and cholesterol; BECAUSE THAT WAS WHAT I WAS TRAINED TO DO! I guess I thought the reason my HDL was low and blood pressure was high was because I was deficient in medication.

Oh yeah, I continued on the low fat, low cholesterol diet plan until I read *Protein Power*. After reading the first few chapters of *Protein Power*, and armed with my biochemical knowledge, I knew for a fact I had told thousands (at that point in my career, probably tens of thousands) of people to eat the wrong way.

Well, after finishing the book, I began a totally different, unaccepted and controversial diet plan. Before I had even changed my diet to the correct one, I knew it was going to work. How did I know it was going to work, you may ask? Because of the biochemistry involved. You see, along with reading *Protein Power*, I also opened the latest copies of my undergraduate and medical books on biochemistry and cellular physiology.

The contents of and the basis for *Protein Power's* claims have been known and printed for years. For years. Oh my goodness!!!! How could I have been so ignorant! Not even has the information been right at arms reach, I HAD READ THE BOOKS! And I wish I could say I only glanced at these textbooks, so that's the reason for my ignorance, but I cannot. Due to my love of biochemistry and cellular physiology, I had read these textbooks cover to cover, AT LEAST 3 TIMES!!!

Am I the embodiment of stupidity? Am I just plain dumb? Nope, I am just a physician trained the way all other physicians have been trained dietarily, and are still being trained in medical schools today.

OK, so let's start a journey together. Come along with me as I take you into the depths of biochemistry and cellular physiology. Now relax. Don't panic. I know the words biochemistry and cellular physiology scare most people into a panic, and perhaps create a sense of impending boredom. You do not need to be frightened and I hope you will not be bored. I will explain biochemistry and cellular physiology to you so you will not only be able to share my story, but understand it too. Once you understand why what I say is true, you will want to change your current eating style, forever.

I will allow you, the reader, to be critical of this book. How can I stop you? I know I said earlier some of my biggest critics will be my colleagues, but that is ok. Their arguments will all be the same. It goes something like 'We all know eating like *that* is dangerous and we do not know the long term ramifications of staying on a diet like *that*."

My only comment will be, "Well, didn't we all *know* that

the world was flat. Hey, some of us even believed in Santa

Claus, and we *knew* that was true."

Was it?

Is it?

OK, let's get started. I have a huge story to tell. And, oh

yeah, don't go and do anything crazy like stop your medi-

cations unless you do so under the guidance of a physician

well versed in this particular style of eating. I don't need a

lawsuit, so don't do it. OK, OK, let's have some fun....

PART I-THE EXPLANATION

CHAPTER ONE –A PRIORI REASONING

Most people's first thought will be "A priori *what,* what the heck does that have to do with a diet book." Well, actually, a lot. A quick glance in any dictionary will define a priori reasoning as a type of deductive reasoning. An inference, say, about what one thinks how things should be. A priori reasoning is based more on theory, than actual experience, as defined in the American Heritage Dictionary, Second Edition.

The problem with a priori reasoning is that it does not always work to explain things. An example of a priori reasoning is the following: it makes perfect sense that when one stands on the beach and looks out at the horizon; the world appears to be flat. So it is very easy to see why for thousands of years we thought the world was flat. But it isn't. We know this for a fact. A priori reasoning was used to come to the incorrect conclusion that the world was flat.

Another problem with a priori reasoning is that you can also use it in silly ways. For instance, to claim the reason a giraffe's neck is long is because its food source is very high. No one would subscribe to this line of reasoning. Would they?

Of course, it is a somewhat complicated task to figure out geometrically that the world is round. Something Galileo Galilei did over three hundred years ago. He actually used accepted geometrical tools of his day to arrive at the correct conclusion about our planet's shape. The interesting thing about Galileo was that he was not congratulated for this truly remarkable achievement; he was placed under house arrest.

PLACED UNDER HOUSE ARREST!!??

For what?!! For proving the truth?!! As a side note do not think for one second that what you are about to read is not as profound as Galileo's proof. (Oh yeah, I like side notes, so I apologize if I get too side notey on you.) The most important thing about Galileo's accomplishment was that it was not arrived at using a priori reasoning.

So what does a priori reasoning have to do with low fat, low cholesterol diet plans? And if you haven't figured it out yet, this book is about why low cholesterol, low fat diets are not only dangerous, but also deadly.

It goes something like this; if the cholesterol or fat in your blood is elevated, it must be because you are eating too much fat and cholesterol. Right? It does make sense when you quickly think about it. This is a priori reasoning and it certainly seems correct.

The problem is that the reason cholesterol and fat become elevated in the blood, is not because one is consuming too much fat or cholesterol in the diet. In fact the opposite is true, which I'll get to later. So that's why a priori reasoning is important to understand. This line of reasoning was used to start the belief (the incorrect belief I may add), that eating cholesterol and fat directly elevates the cholesterol and fat in the blood. And to lower these values one must eat fewer foods containing fat and cholesterol. And this is wrong, but it is still thought to be true, and a priori reasoning lies at the base of these incorrect assumptions.

Just like it was a complicated task to arrive at the correct spherical shape of the earth, it is somewhat of a complicated task to understand why low fat, low cholesterol diets do not work, are dangerous, and will kill you in the end. Complicated yes, but impossible to understand, not at all. And you *will* understand why by the end of this book. Now that wasn't so bad was it? You're actually about to start chapter two. Oh wait, as another side note, do not think for a second that your friendly neighborhood drug companies want you to understand any of this. If people begin to understand, these companies lose money, lots of it.

OK, on to chapter two.

CHAPTER TWO-CHOLESTEROL

Now that we know the reasoning, and I use that term loosely, behind how low cholesterol, low fat diets started; let's examine in a little more detail the substance called cholesterol. We'll look at fats a little later.

Cholesterol is considered a type of fat, a sterol to be precise. Its production starts with sugar molecules. Please read the preceding statement again. Yes, cholesterol production begins when the cells of the body see sugar molecules. These sugar molecules are modified within the cells of the body (predominantly liver cells, but any cell can make cholesterol) with the final product being, yes, cholesterol.

You might ask, "Why would our bodies make such a deadly substance?" Our bodies make cholesterol because our cells, each and every one of them, need cholesterol to survive. Cholesterol is found in our cell's membrane, is the starting point for the production of hormones like testosterone, estradiol, progesterone, cortisol and bile acid salts; and the list goes on. Without cholesterol in our cell's membrane and without the other things we make from cholesterol; we're dead. The cell membrane is what makes a cell, a cell. Without a cell membrane, we have no cells and there's no us. Without the other stuff we make from cholesterol, we could not survive either.

Getting back to how cholesterol is made, I know what you're thinking; "How come I was never told that cholesterol is made from sugar?" How come you were never told that the very foods that DO NOT contain cholesterol are the very foods that the body uses to MAKE cholesterol. It's because doctors, dieticians and nutritionists have forgotten themselves.

For my physician readers (who may be reading this book in the closet and only you know why, everyone else may skip this little side note), remember glycolysis? Come on, I bet you do. Remember the end product of glycolysis, that thing called pyruvate. Does acetyl Co A ring a bell? It should. It comes from the modification of pyruvate during the aerobic metabolism of glucose. Now who out there remembers that when two molecules of acetyl Co A come together it forms acetoacetyl Co A? Huh? Any takers?

OK, this is for extra credit. Does anyone remember that "all twenty seven carbon atoms found in cholesterol come from acetyl CoA?[1] Mevalonate ring a bell. How about squalene? OK, OK I'll stop now. I know. It was embarrassing for me, too, when I came to the realization that I had forgotten how cholesterol is made. But please do not go on thinking that the cholesterol made in the body comes from anything other than the modification of a sugar molecule. This is so utterly important to understand, so crucial, it bears repeating. Cholesterol is made in the body from sugar. It is through the modification of a sugar molecule that we make the majority of cholesterol in our bodies.

Now, to get to cholesterol from sugar molecules requires a review of biochemical pathways, physiological feedback loops (say that three times fast) and a whole bunch of other biochemical mumbo jumbo, which is enough to give anyone a

---

1   *Biochemistry*, Lubert Stryer, Fourth Edition, p.692

headache. That's why I stopped a few paragraphs ago. But don't worry; we'll be reviewing no biochemical pathways here.

Suffice it to say that sugar is the starting point for cholesterol production. So every time you eat something which contains sugar, you are setting in motion the processes that the body needs to make cholesterol.

Now it must be mentioned that the cells of the body produce a greater amount of cholesterol than is consumed by us daily.[2] This means we are producing more cholesterol than we are eating. So let me ask a question, if we want to effectively lower our cholesterol, and I mean effectively, would I modify my dietary intake of cholesterol, or attempt to modify the body's production of cholesterol?

Well, let's think it through. The body makes more cholesterol than I consume. So if I can somehow modify how much cholesterol my body makes, I will effect a greater change on my cholesterol numbers. If I change how much

2 *Textbook of Medical Physiology*, Guyton & Hall, Ninth Edition, p.872

cholesterol I am eating, I will change the number less. But isn't that exactly what we are doing when we change our dietary consumption of cholesterol, by following low fat, low cholesterol diets? By following the accepted diet for reducing cholesterol, you are marginally influencing the cholesterol number.

By lowering your carbohydrate intake (I like the moniker carbs for short, it's the cool way to say it) you are lowering the amount of sugar molecules a cell sees, and if the cell sees less sugar, the cell makes less cholesterol.

As a side note, carbs are broken down into sugars, so whenever one eats carbs, the cell will see sugar.

 Now I mentioned above, and the statement was taken directly from one of the most widely used Medical Physiology textbooks in colleges across America, that it is the body's own production of cholesterol that contributes most to the cholesterol present in our bodies.

Soooo, lets combine some thoughts. By lowering your carb intake, the cell sees less sugar, less sugar means less cholesterol production by our cells, and voila; you just altered the most important contributor to cholesterol production in the body. Yes, it's that simple. So simple, it's embarrassing. But wait, it gets even more embarrassing (maybe I should have titled the book-Much To My Chagrin, or Embarrassed; nah Genocide's more shocking and, unfortunately, truthful).

Ok, so some people may be wondering what happens when we eat cholesterol. After all, doctors are taught that it's the cholesterol we eat which gets us in trouble. Are you sitting down? I hope so; because here's the kicker. When we eat cholesterol our body actually diminishes its production of cholesterol. Huh? Do you mean to tell me that when I eat cholesterol my body actually slows down its production of cholesterol? Yup, it's true.

So let's put some more ideas together. The low cholesterol diet means more whole grains (carbs), fruits (carbs) and vegetables (carbs), and obviously less cholesterol. Guess what you just did. You just set in motion all the body needs TO MAKE MORE CHOLESTEROL!!!! Can I hear a great big OOOPPPS!!!!

It's the classic negative biofeedback loop that makes this happen. When one ingests cholesterol, since it's a fat, it can transfuse right through the cell and nuclear membranes. Eventually it binds with the actual DNA of the cell and turns off the production of the enzymes that make cholesterol. Specifically, the production of the enzyme 3-hydroxy-3-methylglutaryl CoA reductase is significantly lowered. Since this is one of the most important enzymes for cholesterol formation, turning off the production of this enzyme, will decrease the production of cholesterol in our bodies.

So that is why low cholesterol diets do not work to significantly lower the level of cholesterol in the blood. Going through it one more time, when we eat carbs, and since the majority of cholesterol in our blood is produced by the body; we provide the cells with what they need to make more cholesterol. And then by lowering cholesterol consumption this sends the message to our body to make more cholesterol. This is because our cells, when they see less cholesterol, will make more of that enzyme mentioned above (3-hydroxy-3-

methylglutaryl CoA reductase). Then more cholesterol will be made. I refer to this as the double whammy effect.

Now you physician readers may be feeling a little uneasy, because I have not mentioned that lowering one's intake of cholesterol in the diet, will oftentimes lower the cholesterol number in the blood stream. Yes, this does happen, but we do not see a significant lowering of the cholesterol number. In fact, in a perfect body, and well who would that be; you only get a lowering of about fifteen percent. So if your cholesterol is, say, 300, which is not an uncommon number to see; by dramatically reducing the cholesterol in your diet, you can possibly (and usually not) lower the number from 300 to 255. For most people, this would not have lowered the cholesterol number enough, and guess what? Now your doctor is reaching for medication to help lower the cholesterol number more.

I often times will say to my patients and colleagues, who never seem to understand my reasoning, because either they do not want to, or truly just don't understand, that if the dietary contribution to your cholesterol number is only fifteen percent, what contributes the other eighty five percent? Well, it's what your body makes of course. So wouldn't it make sense to try to modify my body's production of cholesterol, since this contributes more to the cholesterol number? Of course! This makes perfect sense, but by starting yourself on a low cholesterol diet, and by eating more carbs, and you have to eat more carbs, because that's all that's left, again, you set in motion all the things the body needs to make more cholesterol. OK, I think I've said enough about cholesterol, and we will talk more about it later. Remember, some people will question what I've written in this chapter, possibly challenging what I say as untrue, but it is not. All one has to do is go to any biochemistry text and read the part on how we make cholesterol, to see that what I say is a fact.

You can take a break if you wish before we get to the next chapter, where we will talk about that scary fat (which is not really all that scary) the triglyceride (said with a rising fiendish, menacing, guttural tone).

CHAPTER THREE-TRIGLYCERIDES

One of the easiest things I do in my practice is lower tri-glycerides, and I do this through diet and diet alone. It is only when somebody doesn't listen to what I tell them to do that I have to resort to the use of medication. But what exactly is a triglyceride and how do I lower this thing so easily? Well, let me tell you.

A triglyceride, as the name suggests, has three glycerides. Get it? Tri means three and the word glyceride follows, so a **tri**-glyceride, has three glycerides. Glyceride is a fancy way of saying fat. So a triglyceride is three fats stuck to-gether. When your doc orders a lipid profile, the triglyc-eride number will be there as well. If your triglyceride reading is high, it means the fats in your blood are high.

Now remember a priori reasoning, it goes something like this; if your triglycerides, or fats in the blood are high, it must be because you are eating too much fat. Right? Well, actually, it's wrong. Dead wrong, with emphasis on the dead. Because that's exactly where you'll wind up if you believe that. And, yes, by the way, most docs still tell their patients to start a low fat diet if their triglycerides are elevated; AND THIS DOES NOT WORK, NEVER, EVER, EVER!!!

Are you ready for this one, the reason the triglycerides elevate in the bloodstream is because of the consumption of carbs. So when you go and start a low fat, low cholesterol diet, again, you will be eating more carbs. We learned in the last chapter this sets up the body to make more cholesterol, but it also allows the body to make more triglycerides as well, That's right, may I hear another great big OOPPPS!!

So putting all this together, eating more whole grains and fruits and less cholesterol, will help to elevate both the cholesterol and triglyceride numbers in the bloodstream, exactly the opposite of what we are trying to accomplish. But exactly *how* does the consumption of carbs elevate the triglyceride number; let's take a look.

When we eat carbs, they are broken down into sugars. Guess what the starting point for the making of a triglyceride is? Hmmm? Yup, you got it, it's sugar. So our bodies make triglycerides from sugar and our bodies make cholesterol from sugar. OK, let's think about this; *the very things that do not contain any fat or cholesterol, are the very things our body uses to make fat and cholesterol.*

By eating more whole grains (carbs) and fruits (carbs), we are providing the body with the very things it needs to make more fat and cholesterol. Yes, I am repeating myself a lot, but I cannot over emphasize how dangerous it is to follow a low fat, low cholesterol diet, as well as eating more whole grains and fruits. This is exactly what the body needs to make all the bad stuff.

It is so frustrating for me to see a patient, who tells me they are on a low fat, low cholesterol diet and that they have been on it for years. They come in and tell me that despite the fact they are eating healthy, they still need to take meds and are having a difficult time losing weight. OF COURSE THEY ARE! What they are essentially doing is giving the body everything it needs to make all the bad things they are trying to lower. But when I attempt to explain this to them, they always go back to the old "Well, all my other doctors before told me to get on a low fat, low cholesterol diet, so I did; and now you are telling me that's wrong, when all the other docs say it's right? What makes you so much smarter."

Of course, during this exchange with my patients, I'm always thinking that, no, I'm not much smarter. Actually, I feel like an idiot for not figuring this out sooner. But what does that say about the majority of physicians who are still telling their patients to start low fat, low cholesterol diets. In fact, just a few minutes ago (I am telling this story to you between seeing my patients), I received a consultative report from a cardiologist who recommended to a patient of mine to start a low fat, low cholesterol diet. Yes, very frustrating.

Another interesting side note is that when patients are told to start low fat, low cholesterol diets, most of you do. But guess what? Most docs don't *believe* you when you tell them you have been on a low fat, low cholesterol diet. You know why? Because when the vast majority of you go for your repeat labs in three to four months, the lipid profile has only changed marginally, if at all. And a lot of the lab reports come back worse.

So you go in to see your physician for the follow up visit, to discuss your latest labs, and when you tell the doc you have been on their prescribed diet, you get the look. You know, the look. From above the glasses, which I find obnoxious, and with that condescending tone you hear "*Sure you have been on the diet.*"

But guess what, you were on the diet. I know it, you know it, but your doc thinks you are lying to them. You know why they think you are lying? Because many times the numbers are worse, not better, and since the doc knows, just absolutely knows, low fat, low cholesterol is the way to go; there's no way your numbers got worse if you were on the diet. But that's exactly why your numbers got worse in the first place: BECAUSE YOU WERE ON THEIR LOW FAT, LOW CHOLESTEROL DIET AND THEY JUST DON'T GET IT!!!!

Why? I told you why; because doctors are not trained to really think, really truly think about things in medical school. We are trained early on in medical school just to accept from the medical community that what they say is true. So that's why it took me so long to wake up and that's why, unfortunately, most docs are still ignorant of this simple truth. Especially for the newly indoctrinated graduates from medical school and even more so, for the Chiefs and Heads of Departments in medical schools and hospitals, you all need to change your way of thinking. Try to get through to those thick craniums. Unfortunately, it isn't going to happen anytime soon. But these are the docs we all look up to for answers; and if they don't know, and worse, if they don't realize they don't know, we are all in trouble. Can you see the problem?

All right, I'm getting myself all worked up; let's get back to the triglyceride. So triglyceride production starts with sugar. I mentioned in chapter two something called glycolysis. This is where the production of cholesterol begins, but fat production can start here too. The sugar molecule is modified and out comes this thing called pyruvate, which is modified again and we get right back to good ole acetyl Co A.

Acetyl Co A, wait a minute, wasn't that the thing that cholesterol was derived from. You got it. So every time you eat sugar (carbs), the sugar will be modified to acetyl Co A, and now you are well on your way to making more fat and cholesterol. Congratulations. Now your doc can put you on meds and the drug companies can pay for their Leer jets.

So now some of you may be wondering, well, hey, "What happens when I eat fat?" Great question, let's see.

Fat digestion occurs in the small intestine. When fat is broken down, it is broken down into its multiple components. Now, this transformed fat will diffuse into your intestinal cells and will be reformed into substances known as chylomicrons. I know my readers who have taken biology will hear a bell ringing. These new fat things will enter a circulatory system known as the lymph.

As a side note, we have two circulatory systems, a closed one and an open one. The closed one you know as your arteries, capillaries and veins, the open circulatory system is referred to as lymph. This is the whitish watery stuff you see when you just barely scrape your hands or knees.

These chylomicrons, which are really just transformed fat, now circulate into an area called the thoracic duct, and empty into veins. Thus becoming part of the regular circulatory system, by entering the bloodstream. These chylomicrons now diffuse into fat cells, liver cells and just about every cell of the body. Whether these are stored or used for fuel depends upon whether carbohydrates are present. In the presence of carbohydrates, the chylomicrons will be stored. If there exists a low amount of carbs in the diet, the fats will be used for energy.

Yes, that's right, our bodies do use fat for fuel. But we will only use fat for fuel if there is no carbohydrate lying around. Fats are pretty tricky, not as straightforward as cholesterol. That's because sometimes fats can be used to make cholesterol, too. But this only happens when carbs are present. If one is following a diet with more fat and cholesterol (notice I did not use the term, high) and low carbs (notice I did not say no carbs), the body will use fat for fuel, cholesterol will be converted to very useful substances, and there will be no extra carbs around to make any more fat or cholesterol, as described above.

There is this myth which has been propagated that the body prefers to use sugar for energy. This is not true. Guyton's Textbook of Medical Physiology states, "Almost all the normal energy requirements of the body can be provided by oxidation of the transported free fatty acid without using any carbohydrate or protein." What this statement means is that the body can use free fatty acids, that is, a single triglyceride, for fuel. It is also widely claimed that our brain cells prefer carbs for fuel. Again, this is wrong. Our brains prefer to use molecules called ketone bodies for its energy source. Interestingly enough, the byproduct of free fatty acid breakdown is ketone bodies. Hmmmm.

So let's put this all together. When we eat fat, it is transformed, pretty quickly I might add, to another fat, which finds its way into our cells. It will be stored or used for fuel, all depending on the presence of carbs. Have a high carb presence and not only will the fat be stored, but we'll. make cholesterol out of it as well. Low carb presence means the fat will be used for fuel, thus leaving very little for storage or cholesterol production. So again, low fat, low cholesterol dieting is NOT the way to go. Unless, of course, you want to gain weight and make more cholesterol and get fat. Yeah, I didn't think so.

CHAPTER FOUR-HDL:
THE GOOD CHOLESTEROL

HDL is a type of cholesterol. HDL stands for High Density Lipoprotein. It is often referred to as the good cholesterol. There are tricks to remember this, such as, let the H in HDL, stand for Healthy or High. So when one sees HDL they'll hopefully remember either healthy or high, and this should remind you that it's the healthy kind and we want this number to be high.

When one goes for the classic lipid profile the HDL will be reported as a number. If one's HDL is less than forty, one is said to have a higher risk of heart disease. Values greater than fifty-nine are viewed as giving one a lower risk of heart disease. Values between forty and fifty-eight are a middle ground where risk could be high or low, depending on other risk factors. These risk factors could be obesity, smoking, high blood pressure or being male. So if having an elevated HDL protects us from CAD (coronary artery disease), the question now becomes; how does one elevate HDL and what exactly is an HDL molecule?

As an extremely important side note male patients greater than forty-five years of age and especially patients male or female at or greater than fifty years of age, who have any underlying medical problems absolutely need nuclear stress tests. A nuclear stress test is where a nuclear isotope is injected into the bloodstream. The patient runs on a treadmill, the heart is monitored while on the treadmill and then monitored again after the running is complete. This is an indirect assessment of potential blockages in the coronary arteries. It needs to be mentioned that even a nuclear stress test can miss coronary artery occlusions, and even a negative stress test, that is, a stress test that does not reveal any blockages, could be falsely negative. What this means is that there are blockages in the coronary arteries, but the nuclear stress test missed it. The only way around this is to perform cardiac catheterizations on everyone and to just stop performing nuclear stress tests since they can sometimes be misleading. I do not recommend performing cardiac catheterizations instead of stress tests as the catheterizations are invasive and have higher complications associated with their performance. Getting a nuclear stress is still the preferred way to indirectly assess for the presence of coronary artery disease. If the stress test is positive, then one needs a cardiac catheterization.

Before I leave this side-note, if you are someone with diabetes and you are a male or female at or greater than fifty years of age, you absolutely need a nuclear stress test. This is because diabetics are notorious for having what is known as silent heart attacks and even blockages, which cause no symptoms whatsoever. You could be walking around with significant CAD and not even know it. And the only chance of knowing this is through a nuclear stress test. I cannot tell you how many times a diabetic patient over the age of fifty has come to see me for a regular check-up, has had no symptoms of chest pain, difficulty in breathing, or any other symptom which might have alerted me to the existence of coronary artery occlusion; has had normal looking

EKGs; I perform a nuclear stress test and find significant coronary artery blockages. The scary thing is that some of these patients had actually been seeing other docs, including cardiologists, who failed to perform a routine nuclear stress test. The bottom line is that if you have diabetes, or any other medical issue, and you are at or greater than the age of fifty, you need a nuclear stress test. If you cannot walk for whatever reason, there are other nuclear stress tests which can be performed to help assess for the presence of CAD. And lastly, if you are male or female at or greater than the age of sixty-YOU ABSOLUTELY NEED A NUCLEAR STRESS TEST NO MATTER WHAT!!!! This is because as we get older we can accrue plaques in our coronary arteries just from being on the planet longer. Now, let's get back to our discussion as to what an HDL molecule is made up of.

First, we'll look at what comprises an HDL molecule. Well, HDL stands for high-density lipoprotein. So, it has to have some protein in it, lipo means fat, so fats there too, and it's high density; but, still, what does *that* mean. It simply means it's a molecule, which contains cholesterol, fat, and protein. Since there's a lower amount of fat in an HDL molecule it's called high density because fat is less dense than protein and cholesterol. The more fat the lower the density, the less fat the higher the density.

OK, now here's something very interesting. Ask your typical internist, family doc, pediatrician, cardiologist, or just about anyone who thinks they know something about HDL, how to increase the HDL in the bloodstream. We all see low HDLs and we see them a lot. Usually in men, but also in women. The answer is almost always the same; if you want to increase your HDL, lower your fat and cholesterol intake and increase your whole grains, fruits and vegetables. This, the above docs say, will increase your HDL.

From our discussion thus far you know immediately your body will have all the things necessary to make more fat and cholesterol. But what *kind* of fat and cholesterol will we make? The fat part is easy; we'll make more triglycerides (you know what, I'm getting tired of spelling out triglycerides so for now on I'm calling them TGs). As far as cholesterol is concerned, again, what kind of cholesterol will we make when we eat a diet low in fat and cholesterol?

Well, cholesterol is cholesterol is cholesterol, so the short answer is; just plain ole cholesterol is formed. But is it HDL, LDL, VLDL or IDL, which I will now call the DLs? Guess what, if you focus on those three letter cholesterols you start to forget that they are simply carrier molecules of cholesterol. That's right, all these DLs carry cholesterol around in the body and exchange it with other DLs. So viewing cholesterol as a good or bad type of cholesterol totally confuses the picture.

Another side note: HDL is known for carrying away cholesterol after a cell dies. After the HDL molecule picks this cholesterol up, it shuttles it away and gives it to other DLs. But why is it considered the good cholesterol? Well, that's because HDL is also known to take cholesterol back to the liver for its removal from the bloodstream

Now the confusing part begins. Exactly how do our bodies actually get rid of cholesterol? There are certain medications that are referred to as bile acid sequestrants. Bile is a substance the liver makes, stores in the gallbladder, and is released to help with the digestion of fats and cholesterol. Bile acid itself contains cholesterol, so the drug companies developed a med which binds with these bile acids, doesn't let them go, and when you poop, out comes the cholesterol. Pretty clever.

Only thing is, these specific types of meds can only lower the cholesterol number by a small amount. Anyone with a high cholesterol number will need another med, assuming the proper diet is not revealed to the patient, to help lower the cholesterol number further. It may appear as if we've come off our topic of HDL, but we really have not.

You would think that if HDL was a good cholesterol it would somehow get rid of the cholesterol from the body, so it couldn't bind to our arteries and kill us. But this does not happen. HDL quickly takes and gives its cholesterol to other DLs. One of which is the LDL transporter, which everyone mistakenly believes is the bad cholesterol. But if HDL is quickly giving its cholesterol to LDL, I'm still confused; wouldn't that make HDL a bad cholesterol too, since it's aiding and abetting the LDL cholesterol? I will discuss more about LDL cholesterol below, but for now understand that LDL is considered the bad cholesterol.

OK, so let's get back to our typical internist, family doc, pediatrician, or cardiologist. When we ask them how to raise the HDL they'll answer exercise, follow a low fat, low cholesterol diet, which means we need to eat more whole grains, fruits and veggies. After sixteen years of practicing medicine I can tell you that this doesn't work. Some docs will be thinking that, "Of course it works." And my reply is that in sixteen years of caring for patients I have rarely seen this diet/exercise approach work to significantly elevate the HDL.

Well, what have I seen work, you might ask ? The only thing I have seen work to substantially increase HDL, doubling it, sometimes increasing the HDL by two and a half times its value; is increasing one's consumption of fat and cholesterol, coupled with a dramatic lowering of one's carb intake.

That's right, as crazy as it sounds, increasing one's consumption of fat and cholesterol in the diet will substantially raise your HDL values. This process can take up to a year, but it works and it works every time. *Every time!* When patients of mine increase their fat and cholesterol consumption their HDLs oftentimes double. *That's right, double!* The best the drug companies can offer is somewhere around a thirty-five percent increase in HDL, but if one increases their consumption of fats and cholesterol and lowers their carb intake, one can increase the HDL by 100%.

To put this in perspective, a thirty-five percent increase means that if your HDL is thirty, not an unusual number to see, the most you can expect as an increase if you're using meds will be from thirty to forty. Sounds impressive until you realize that you are still at increased risk of heart disease even with an HDL in the forty range. How about we take that HDL of thirty and change it into a sixty or seventy, this can be done if you follow the correct diet.

I really am not sure why the HDL doubles. I've read the books, but cannot figure it out. Only thing I can come up with is since the body isn't making as much cholesterol, it chooses to make HDL and the good LDL preferentially over the others. So now one may wonder, what happens to the LDL thing, you know, that thing we doctors mistakenly call the bad cholesterol. I'll show you in Chapter Six. Before we can talk intelligently about LDL, we need to discuss some basic math and I mean really basic math, that is, the math used to calculate all the typical LDLs in our country.

CHAPTER FIVE-THE FRIEDEWALD EQUATION-AN EXTREME DEMONSTRATION IN PHYSICIAN IGNORANCE

There's a show out now called, Are You Smarter Than A 5th Grader? For most docs when it comes to understanding math, I mean really basic math, the overwhelming answer will be no. Let's face it, when most people hear the word math, they cringe, their bellies tighten up, and some of us may even vomit. But I'm not talking about calculus or even algebra. What I'm referring to here is simple addition, subtraction and division. You don't even need to multiply (thank goodness). Let me explain what this equation is and why it's important you understand it.

So what exactly is this Friedewald Equation anyway? In the US when you go to the lab to have your lipid profile checked, there are only three things measured. These are the Total Cholesterol, the HDL and the triglycerides.

These three values are then used to *calculate* the LDL. It is important to realize that the LDL is not measured directly from the blood. This has profound implications when one is trying to interpret the lipid profile.

The equation states that the LDL is equal to the Total Cholesterol minus the HDL and subtracted from this is the triglycerides divided by 5 (see below).

$$\text{LDL (calculated)} = \text{Total Cholesterol} - \text{HDL} - \frac{\text{TG}}{5}$$

So when you give your blood, the numbers of the total cholesterol, the HDL and TGs are placed into the equation, and voila, out comes your LDL. Now look very carefully at how simple this equation is. It is simple, isn't it? What do you notice? There's a lot of subtraction going on and one fraction. This fraction is important because as you divide the same number into a lower number, what do you think happens? For instance, divide one hundred by five. You get twenty of course. Now divide fifty, a lower number, by five. Now we get ten. So dividing a lower number by the same number results in a LOWER number. It's quite simple.

This lower number is particularly important because it is being subtracted from another part of the equation. So what happens if you subtract a lower number from something? Unless you are dealing with negative integers, you will get a HIGHER number. As an example, subtract five from ten. The result is five. Now subtract two, a lower number from ten, and eight is the result. Eight is higher than five. Still not tricky.

Now let's digress a little and talk about what the total cholesterol really means. We have not done this yet and it really is quite simple. The total cholesterol is just that, the total cholesterol. We arrive at the total cholesterol by adding together the HDL, LDL (remember the LDL is calculated here, not measured) and the VLDL (for some reason the IDL does not even get honorable mention). So the equation looks like this:

$$\text{Total Cholesterol} = \text{HDL} + \text{LDL} + \text{VLDL}; \text{ where VLDL} = \frac{\text{TG}}{5}$$

Now, what do you think happens to the total cholesterol if you increase, say, the LDL? That's right, the total goes up. What about if the VLDL increases? Uh huh, the total goes up. Wait a minute. What if the HDL goes up? Bingo, so too will the total cholesterol.

As a very, very important side note, this is why when one begins to lower their carbs and to eat more fat and cholesterol the total cholesterol may increase. So it is very important NOT to panic. A very common scenario is the following; a patient figures out that the right way to eat is to eat less carbs and to eat more fat, protein, and cholesterol. They go for their lab work and their doc notices that while the HDL went up dramatically, the total cholesterol went up too. Then the patient is admonished against what they did. They are told those diets are bad for you. Then they are told to start a low fat, low cholesterol diet and guess what; when they check their numbers out in a few months they are so bad they wind up on cholesterol lowering meds.

This is an absolute tragedy. The physician who advises their patient to abandon a low carb, more fat, more cholesterol, more protein diet because the total cholesterol went up, but so, too, did the HDL; is demonstrating extreme ignorance of what total cholesterol is all about. This should never happen, but yet it happens every day. Every single day in almost all the physician's offices all over the world. But wait, it gets even worse.

Remember I said it is important to know that LDL is calculated, not measured. The reason this is important is because when the HDL goes up the total cholesterol may go up. And when the TGs go down you wind up subtracting a smaller number from the rest of the equation. Well, look at the equation. What will happen to your total cholesterol when you raise your HDL? That's right, it will go up. Again, look at the equation. What do you think you will get when you subtract a higher HDL from a higher total cholesterol? And remember, the total cholesterol is higher because the HDL is higher. Let's do some math together to figure it out.

Subtract thirty-five, a common HDL to see, from, say, a total cholesterol of two hundred thirty. You get one hundred ninety five. Now subtract fifty, a pretty common rise to see when you're eating the correct way, from a total cholesterol of two hundred sixty five. We now get two hundred fifteen. Do some more to prove it to yourself. The point, to say it again, is that when we subtract a higher number from a higher number, we wind up with a higher number. Now when we subtract a smaller number from this higher number, the result will be a higher number. The smaller number we are subtracting results from the TGs being lower when we lower our carb intake and eat more fat and cholesterol. And from the above discussion, we have seen that when we divide a lower number by the same number, the result is a lower number. It is this lower number we are subtracting from the higher number we arrived at above.

So the end result to the calculated LDL value when your total cholesterol and HDL go up and your triglycerides go lower, IS THAT THE LDL GOES HIGHER BECAUSE OF THE WAY IT IS CALCULATED! We want the HDL to go higher. We want the fats in your blood to be lower. When this happens it will oftentimes raise the LDL. No, it doesn't happen in everyone, but it happens in just about everyone and it is solely due to the way the LDL is calculated.

Now guess what happens when you walk into your doc's office after spending three months eating the way you should. Your HDL will be higher, which is great, but this may make the total cholesterol increase. Your triglycerides will be lower, which is awesome because that's what you want. But your LDL will be higher. Again, based on the formula the lab uses to calculate the LDL, the LDL will be higher when your HDL is higher and your TGs are lower. When your doctor reads your lab report do you really think that she or he is going to say, "Wow, great, everything's fantastic!" Not a chance. All your doc sees is an elevated total cholesterol and an elevated LDL. They panic, your doctor that is, and immediately want to place you on cholesterol lowering meds. But wait a minute; if they are so interested in lowering the calculated LDL we can do this by raising your TGs or lowering your HDL: exactly what we don't want to do.

Just to bring everyone up to date. I think the latest guidelines say to keep the LDL below seventy if you have risk factors for heart disease. I have difficulty with this concept because we are using the calculated LDL, not measuring it directly. Sure, the cholesterol lowering meds work, but all too often I see well trained cardiologists freaking out because they can't get the calculated LDL below seventy, or even one-hundred for that matter. And they'll just keep pushing the dose higher and higher and higher. If they just stopped and thought the process through they would realize that in the vast majority of people this approach will not work. Why? Because their patient's TGs may be low and their HDLs may be where they should be, so based on the calculation, the LDL will never get below 70.

But one cannot really harp on these docs for what they are doing. They are simply doing what they were trained to do. They apply the guidelines, do not think for themselves, and they push the accepted medications for the treatment of cholesterol. But this would still be defined as ignorance, wouldn't it? And whom do we blame for the millions of people who die each year because of this?

The lipid profile numbers that we should be paying attention to are the HDL and TGs only. What I like to use is the TG to HDL ratio. Keep this ratio at or under two and you're sitting pretty. If it rises above two, be careful, because now not only are you looking at an increased risk of heart disease, but also diabetes and cancer. Two other diseases we will be discussing shortly.

Now on to chapter six.

CHAPTER SIX- CALORIES

This topic really burns me up. Get it, burns me up...OK, sorry. I couldn't resist. So who can tell me what a calorie is? Any takers? Give up? All right, a calorie is the amount of heat needed to raise the temperature of one gram of water by one degree in the Celsius scale. This definition is referenced and repeated in numerous scientific and medical textbooks. Now the next question I ask is, "What the heck does this have to do with human nutrition?"The short answer is absolutely nothing. Now the longer answer.

It seems that wherever you turn someone is harping on the calorie. Calorie this and calorie that. Lower your caloric intake and you'll lose weight. Increase your calories and stop exercising and you'll gain weight. I am here to tell you that this is simply false.

Over the last nine years of starting my patients on low carb, more fat, more cholesterol and more protein diets,

I have seen HDLs double, type 2 diabetics cured, blood pressures that were once difficult to control become normal, thousands of pounds lost, TGs lowered to normal; all this while usually *increasing* the caloric intake.

I actually had one patient who went from consuming 2000 calories a day to eating 6000-8000 calories a day and while keeping his exercise regimen the same, LOST WEIGHT. That's right, he increased his caloric intake, did not increase his exercise level, and lost weight. This seems to defy the senses. My patient did not understand it. I did not understand it because I was ignorant. Then I did what very few doctors even dare to do. I started to think for myself. And I figured out why using the calorie as a dietary guide is a waste of time.

I defined what a calorie is above. But how do we go about determining how many calories are in, say, a burger, or a piece of lettuce. When we buy a food product at the supermarket there's nutritional information on the side-packaging label. One of the first things we are told to look for is 'how many calories are there per serving.' So we look and we see how many calories there are.

But I still haven't answered the question as to how we actually measure calories. Well it's really quite simple. What we do is we take the food item we wish to measure and burn it in a closed container. This container is filled with water and also has a thermometer in it. We watch how many degrees change on the thermometer and each degree change represents a calorie. So for instance, if we burn a quarter pound of meat in this container (called a calorimeter, by the way), and the temperature goes up two hundred degrees, that represents two hundred calories. Generally only a single food item is burned. But one can burn the whole, say, quarter pounder with cheese, and see what the degree change is; thus arriving at how many calories existed in that particular food item.

The problem with the calorie is that this measurement occurs in a closed system. A closed system is one where we know everything that is happening within that system. And I mean everything. For instance, I know what the thing weighs that I'm burning; I know the size of the container I'm using; I know the starting and ending temperature on the thermometer; I know how much water is in the container, and so on.

Now, our bodies are not closed systems, they are open systems. This means we have only a general idea of what happens when we eat, say, a quarter pounder. So what happens when we eat a quarter pound of meat? Well, first we need to chew this food and then swallow it. It gets to the stomach where the digestive process continues. When the meat leaves the stomach and enters the small intestine, this is where the problems start.

When the quarter pound of meat finds its way into the first part of the small intestine (known as the duodenum), pandemonium begins. A bunch of enzymes and hormones are released from the pancreas and small intestine, bile is secreted from the gallbladder to help with digestion, and all of these enzymes interact in such a complex way that we are still trying to figure out what's going on. If any of you doctors think we, as physicians, understand the whole digestive process, all I can say is sitagliptin.

For my non-physician readers I apologize, but I need to make a point, to underscore the continued ignorance of us docs. For my docs, please do not take offence, and don't confuse ignorance with stupidity. Stupidity is difficulty in understanding a topic, and I do not like the word at all. Ignorance occurs when we really, truly, honestly just don't know because we just haven't been smart enough to discover something yet.

OK, so I said sitagliptin. This is a new medication for type 2 diabetics only. It is a dipeptidyl-peptidase 4-enzyme inhibitor. This newly discovered entity works by interfering with certain things secreted by the intestine. No, this is not the part of the book where I lose everyone. I'm just trying to make a point. We docs only found out about this over the last few years and we had no idea how important this thing was in sugar regulation. So for anyone who thinks we know it all by now, especially with digestion, you're sadly mistaken because we've only just uncovered the proverbial tip of the iceberg.

So getting back to where we were, there is no way to exactly measure anything other than the weight of what

you ate. That's it. Once we swallow the food so many complex things occur, there is absolutely no way to keep track
of everything that happens during the digestive process.

So let's put everything together. Closed system versus
open system. In a closed system we know everything, and
I mean everything that is happening. In the open system we
know very little, as there are so many different variables.
So my problem with the calorie is that it is only useful if
you want to know how much heat will be generated from
the food you ate. That's it.

Not to sound silly but when we eat food, the food doesn't
just go into the belly and get burned up and that's it.
Humans do not *burn* food, we *digest* it. To say there's four
hundred calories in a food item disregards the fact and I
mean fact, that the calorie only tells us how much heat will
be given off when you burn the food, in a closed, regulated
environment.

I ask again, "What does the calorie have to do with human
nutrition?' And my answer remains the same--Nothing.
That is why when many of my patients increase their caloric

intake, which we know now means nothing anyway, they lose weight. This is because they are eating foods which encourage the whole fat burning process. And when you put into motion the fat burning process, not only are you not storing fat, but also you're not making cholesterol, your blood pressure lowers, and your blood sugars normalize. But these are subjects for other chapters.

If, on the other hand, one eats carbs, now you'll set into motion all the body needs to make all the bad stuff. It just so happens that one-gram of carbs and protein contain four calories, whereas one gram of fat contains nine calories. This is why we're told to avoid fat because it has more calories than carbs and protein per gram. The reasoning is that if we eat fat we ingest more calories to burn as opposed to the consumption of carbs and protein. And then, the argument continues, you will get fatter by eating the fat, again, because it contains more calories.

As a side note, notice that whenever we talk about calories we use the word 'burn'. Like, since you ate all that fat, now you have to 'burn' it off. Or, I ate so much when I was on vacation; I have to 'burn' it off. Well, where do you think this term 'burn' is derived from? Exactly, from the same way we determined the calorie in the first place; we 'burned' the stuff in the container.

So, when I'm in the examining room with my patients and the term calorie comes up, I immediately tell them that the calorie is irrelevant. I tell them that a calorie measurement is only useful if you want to know how much heat is given off when you burn something. I also add that our bodies do not work that way, we do not burn, we digest. I explain about the calorimeter and tell them this container burns things, it doesn't digest like we do. And the final thing I say is that if "I were king for a day, I would eliminate the term calorie from all the side packaging information labels." What would I put there? How many carbs, protein, fat, cholesterol, vitamins, minerals, fiber, sugar alcohols (which we'll talk about later), and to list the presence or absence of trans fats (which we'll talk about later as well).

CHAPTER SEVEN-SUGAR IS
SUGAR IS SUGAR

Sugar is very important to discuss. I have already mentioned sugar a bunch of times. I have already shared the biggest secret that fat and cholesterol production starts with sugar. So now let's really learn about sugar.

We all have heard of sugar. It comes in many varieties. There are your simple sugars like glucose (the most popular) and fructose (found in fruit). Then you have the weirder ones like galactose, xylose, allose, and ribose. The big fancy way to refer to these sugars is by calling them monosaccharides since they only consist of a single sugar molecule. Some of these you may have heard of, others even your doctor has never heard of.

Now there are your more complex types of sugars where two sugars are attached to one another. The three most common are sucrose (table sugar), lactose (found in milk) and maltose. These sugars need to be broken down before our body can use them. They are referred to as disaccharides, with the di referring to the fact there are two sugar molecules attached to one another.

Let's talk a little bit about carbs and where they fit in. Carbs are basically glucose molecules all strung together like beads on a string. A single bead would represent a single glucose molecule. Sometimes these string beads are short. Sometimes there are millions of beads on a string.

Before we can use the glucose in a long string the string would need to be broken down into its single beads or glucose molecules. After the body has done this, the glucose may now be treated in different ways. If there is an overabundance of glucose in the system, as is often the case, the glucose will be stored first in the liver and then in muscles. After the liver and muscles have their fill the glucose molecule will be used to make cholesterol and TGs, and the extra TGs will be stored as fat on our bodies. It doesn't take long to fill up our livers and muscles with glucose. Since it doesn't take long to fill up our livers and muscles, and since most people eat more glucose then they should, there is plenty of sugar left over to make cholesterol, TGs and to store as fat.

The current recommendation for carbohydrate intake is somewhere between two hundred to two hundred fifty grams of carbohydrates per day. No one, and I mean no one, should be consuming this amount of carbs in their diet. Obesity, heart disease, diabetes, and cancer (and I will discuss the link between carbs and cancer later) are being seen more and more in our society. We are even seeing, in children younger than ten, what were once thought to be diseases of adults; that is, obesity and diabetes.

Most of the medical profession is scratching their heads trying to figure out why this is so. The answer sadly enough is right before their eyes, but the medical physicians just cannot see it We have more and more people on low fat, low cholesterol diets and this includes our children. When we follow a low fat. low cholesterol diet, we **must** consume more carbs. As we consume more carbs we send all the signals to our body to get fat and make more cholesterol.

Eating less cholesterol sends the signal to make more cholesterol. We are shortening the life expectancy of our children by the continuous propagation of the low cholesterol, low fat diet.

To me, being a part of the medical profession that is promulgating this deadly diet is embarrassing. Why is it that more docs have not figured out that when one follows a low fat, low cholesterol diet, they wind up less healthy then when they started?

Why?

Again, it's because we are not trained to think for ourselves in medical school. We are told to just listen and leave all the thinking to the specialists, or the doctors on the *special* committees.

Unfortunately, it is these specialists or committee members who are the blindest. They continue to espouse low fat, low cholesterol diets, continue to tell us that eating whole grains and fruits are good for you, and continue to mistakenly believe that it is a lack of physical exercise which is the main contributor to the obesity epidemic.

This is just plain wrong. Why is it that I have had many cases where I've dealt with morbidly obese patients, who I start on a low carb diet, who lose significant amounts of weight *before they even start* an exercise regimen? Yes, these patients start to lose weight and lots of it, *before they start exercising*. If what the experts say is true this should not be happening. But it does, every single day in my practice.

Now don't get me wrong. I am not saying exercise is not important. It is and it is very important. It does accelerate weight loss when done correctly. But to tell a patient with knee pain to start walking when they are three hundred pounds is negligent. How about we take some weight off, say, fifty pounds and then have them start walking. This way there is less stress and strain on the hips, knees and ankles when they start walking. This just makes sense to me. OK, I digressed again, let's get back to our discussion of sugar.

Another huge problem is that our medical professionals would like you to believe that the same sugar molecules are somehow different. For instance, that if the sugar molecule is from fruit, it is natural and that's OK. Or, if it comes from whole wheat, again, it's natural and that's fine.

Well, I am here to stop that myth. Please remember, sugar is sugar is sugar. Repeat it to yourself a hundred, no wait, a thousand times a day. I tell my patients this all the time. What that means is that a glucose molecule from whole wheat bread is no different than if it came from broccoli, or a snickers bar, or from table sugar, and on and on and on. The fact is when glucose is presented to our cells our cells cannot distinguish where that glucose molecule came from, because all glucose molecules look exactly the same to the cell.

Glucose is no good to us unless it gets inside our cells, which is where all the modifications to it take place. The thing that allows glucose to get into the cell is something called insulin. The pancreas makes insulin and squirts it into our bloodstream every time the pancreas sees sugar. If glucose cannot get into the cell it will remain in the blood-stream. When glucose stays in the bloodstream it begins to attach to the cell's outer surfaces, causing distortions and malfunctioning of organs. This is why diabetics have problems like blindness, need dialysis and may have to have amputations. Again, it's all about the sugar. I will be talking more about diabetes in a later chapter.

To think that our cells can tell where the glucose came from, say from a vegetable or a snickers bar, is ignorant. In order for the cell to do this it would need to be able to know what we ate. And then the cell would have to say to itself, "Ah hah, this glucose molecule came from a snickers bar, so I'm going to do bad things with it." Or, the cell would say, "Alright, this glucose molecule came from broccoli so let's do good things with it." And what would happen if we ate a snickers bar along with broccoli, would our cells be able to tell the difference between the glucose molecules now?

Of course not, but this is exactly what medical professionals suggest when they say snickers bars have bad sugar and broccoli has good sugar. There is no such thing. Sugar is sugar is sugar. And it is all treated the same way when it gets to the cell.

Now don't think for a second I don't care what you are eating sugar wise. I would much prefer the green leafy vegetable to the snickers bar. My point is that when following a low carb diet, *all sugars count*.

One of the most interesting things that started happening when I first started placing patients on low carb diets (and from now on when I say low carb, you probably already figured out I also mean more fat, more cholesterol and more protein) was that they would say they were doing low carb, but their cholesterol and TGs would come back elevated. As a doctor I am unique as I actually listen to, and believe my patients. Most docs would suspect their patients were lying, but I don't until the evidence presents itself to the contrary. Anyway, when the TG and cholesterol numbers came back elevated, I began to ask about everything my patients were eating. No luck, all low carb. I was perplexed and left scratching my head, then, Eureka! I got it.

I was asking them what they were eating, but I wasn't asking them what they were drinking. I know, sounds ignorant on my part and it was. When I began to ask what my patients with the elevated TGs and cholesterol were drinking, it almost always turned out to be some kind of fruit juice. When I asked them to stop drinking the juice I would always get these weird looks. Some would say "What do you mean, everyone knows fruit juice is good for you because it is a *natural* sugar." Guess what happened to the TGs and cholesterol numbers when the juice was stopped. Good guess, you figured out immediately that the TG and cholesterol numbers dropped, sometimes significantly. Here's why.

The sugar in fruit is fructose. It is not too much different in structure when compared to glucose. Fructose is easily changed to glucose by a simple method. (Called isomerization.) Once fructose is changed to glucose, it is treated the same way extra glucose is; it is converted to TGs and cholesterol. So the sugar in the fruits we eat can and will be converted into the very things fruit does not contain, that is, fats and cholesterol. Let's hear another big Oopps!

OK, here's one for you. What would you say if I told you that if you eat a piece of fruit and a snickers bar, the sugar from the fruit will wind up in the fat cells a lot quicker than the sugar in the snickers bar. So we get fatter, quicker, by eating fruit. The reason: because the sugar in the snickers bar, mainly glucose, has to go through the liver before it can get to the fat cell. Since the number one storage fuel molecule in our fat cells is fructose, and since the sugar in fruit is already fructose; no change is needed and the fructose from the fruit goes directly into the fat cell. Yes, we do get fat by eating fruit.

"But Hey," I hear everyone yelling, fruit is natural, so it has to be good. My comment, arsenic and cyanide are natural, but I wouldn't eat them. Ok, maybe a bad comparison, but is it? This so called natural sugar will allow us to get fatter, increase our TGs, lower our HDLs, worsen our diabetes, increase our blood pressure and increase our risk of cancer. And I can go on and on. I tell my patients fruit is a poison, especially to diabetics, and I mean it when I say, don't eat it!

Enough about sugar. Let's talk about something really interesting. Let's talk about what I like to call the dirty little hormone; Insulin.

CHAPTER EIGHT-INSULIN-THE ROOT OF ALL EVIL?

I can make this complicated or I can make this simple. After all, I am a doctor. Since I like to keep things simple, we'll stick to keeping it simple. Ahhh, Insulin, what can I say about insulin that hasn't already been said? Well, actually, a lot.

First off, let me be the first to tell you to be afraid of insulin, be very, very afraid. It is actually insulin that controls how and when sugar will be changed into cholesterol and fat. So the more insulin we secrete, the more cholesterol and fat we make. And as a little aside, insulin also increases our risk of developing and spreading cancer, which I'll explain later. So now you must be wondering, "What is insulin and where does it come from?"

Insulin is referred to as a polypeptide hormone. Hormones come in many shapes and sizes. Some are made up of proteins, others are created from cholesterol. That's right, cholesterol is necessary for the development of many very important hormones. I mentioned this before. Testosterone, estrogen, and cortisol are but a few. Without these hormones, we die. So, without cholesterol, well, I'm sure you get it...

A hormone brings messages that control the activities of our cells. They are very important for normal cellular function. We are taught in biology classes that the main role of insulin is to allow sugar to get into the cell. This is true. Without insulin, sugar has a very difficult time getting into cells.

The pancreas in response to the presence of carbohydrates secretes insulin. So, whenever we eat carbohydrates and/ or food containing sugar, the pancreas will squirt out insulin. Now it is true that one of insulin's roles is to help sugar get into cells; but insulin does a lot more. A whole lot more.

As I started to mention above, it is insulin that controls many of the very important steps which allow our bodies to make cholesterol. Insulin also sends the signals for us to make more triglycerides. And it is the presence of insulin, which prevents us from losing weight.

All doctors know that in medical language insulin is referred to as an anabolic hormone. Anabolic simply means growth promoting. Some of my readers will recognize anabolic as preceding the word steroid, such as anabolic steroids used by athletes. And it means the same thing there; anabolic steroids promote growth.

The reason insulin is anabolic is because, again, it sends all the signals to our body's cells to make fat and to prevent us from losing weight. Insulin controls key enzymes for cholesterol synthesis, most notably HMG CoA reductase (also known as 3-hydroxy-3-methylglutaryl CoA reductase). When insulin is present it will tell this enzyme to make more cholesterol.

Remember insulin is secreted every time we eat carbohydrates (unless you are a Type I diabetic, which I'll discuss a little later). Insulin will then tell the very thing that helps make cholesterol, HMG CoA reductase, to make more cholesterol. Oh yeah, don't forget that our bodies actually use sugar to make cholesterol. So let me make this perfectly clear. Not only by eating carbs are we giving the body what it needs to *make* cholesterol; when the body secretes insulin in response to carbohydrates, the insulin actually speeds up cholesterol production. When we eat carbs we are giving the body everything it needs *to make more cholesterol*.

Now this HMG CoA reductase thing is not just a way for me to show off and say big words. It is very important for cholesterol production. In biochemical language we refer to this enzyme as the rate-limiting step in cholesterol synthesis. This is a fancy way of saying that once this enzyme gets started, it's going to finish what it started doing, and there aint no turning back. So once insulin encourages this enzyme to work, it will make cholesterol no matter what.

For our body's sake it is better that it sees as little insulin as possible. The only way to have any effect on insulin's presence is by lowering the carb intake. That's it. There's no other way to really, truly have an effect on insulin levels in the blood other than by lowering your carb intake.

Lower your insulin level and you lower the activity of that HMG thing. Oh, and something else. Remember when I mentioned a little while ago that eating cholesterol lowers your body's production of cholesterol. Guess how it does it? Well, when you eat cholesterol it actually combines with the HMG CoA reductase and tells it not to work as hard. The cholesterol actually turns off the enzyme that makes itself. But it doesn't stop there. The cholesterol in the foods we eat will also tell the cells, which make cholesterol, to make less of the very enzyme that makes itself.

So eating less carbs helps by not giving the body what it needs to make cholesterol. Lowering the carb intake also means less insulin secretion. Less insulin secretion, less stimulation and production of HMG. Less stimulation and production of HMG, less cholesterol production.

When I place a patient on a low carb diet, I also encourage them to eat more cholesterol, not high, simply more. Let's simplify what happens when we eat cholesterol-containing foods. More cholesterol in the diet, less stimulation and production of HMG. Less stimulation and production of HMG, less cholesterol is made. So, by eating lower carbs and more cholesterol, we make less cholesterol. Period.

What is also very interesting is how the major drugs we docs use to lower cholesterol work. These meds are referred to as statins. The statins actually prevent HMG CoA reductase from working. By doing this these meds lower cholesterol production.

But we can have a similar and more dramatic effect when we lower the carbs and eat more cholesterol. When we eat this way we are manipulating the ability of HMG to make cholesterol and we are also telling the body to stop making HMG. The cholesterol lowering meds do not go this far. They only work on the HMG. With low carbs, we lower cholesterol naturally, and we can avoid medication all together.

Another question, which may come up is, "How does insulin affect the TG number and our fat stores?" Well, when the pancreas in response to a carb meal secretes insulin, the insulin will also interact with the enzymes responsible for fat production and utilization.

"Insulin inhibits lipolysis."[1] This is a statement found in a Biochemistry book I read more than a few times in college. This statement is so very important, yet I did not understand the profoundness of it until nine years ago. What the statement means is that insulin slows down the breakdown of fat in our body. In fact, when insulin is present, our body is sent the signal to not only stop burning fat, but to make more fat. The more insulin, the more difficult it is to lose weight. And weight gain is inevitable the longer insulin is around. What keeps insulin around? Eating carbs. So if you want to make it very difficult to lose weight, eat more carbs. Exactly what we do when we follow a low fat, low cholesterol diet.

Another hormone, glucagon, is also secreted by the pancreas. When this hormone is secreted it has a reverse effect than that of insulin. The more glucagon, the more fat we burn and fat storage is prevented. What causes a release

---

1   *Biochemistry*, Lubert Stryer, Fourth Edition, p.606

of glucagon? Avoidance of carbs and the consumption of protein in the diet.

It might be a good time to re-visit the whole concept of the calorie and why the calorie is irrelevant in human nutrition. Remember we discussed that calories were measured in a closed system, where we knew everything about the system. I also mentioned that our bodies are open systems, where it is impossible with our knowledge today to measure everything that is happening in the body. A great example of this open system concept is glucagon and insulin. Once we eat a food substance, the hormones insulin and glucagon (among many hundreds, thousands? of other hormones and digestive enzymes) are secreted. The interplay between even these two hormones is complex, but just remember this; insulin makes us get fat and stay fat; glucagon sends the signal to use fat and to not gain weight. Eat carbs and insulin is secreted and you get fat; eat less carbs and more protein, less insulin and more glucagon will be secreted, and this helps us lose weight.

There is no way to measure exactly what is happening, that is, how much glucagon was secreted versus how much insulin? Ok, well maybe we can measure in the blood-stream these two hormones, but what about the hundreds of others, what about the digestive enzymes, what about all the things we haven't even discovered yet? I'm getting a headache just thinking about it. Since a calorie is measured in a closed system and our bodies are open systems, again, using the term caloric to help understand any nutritional concept is like comparing apples to kites. They just are not the same. The calorie is *irrelevant*; do not use it, ever. Unless you are a quantitative heat chemist.

We need to get into a little more detail about how insulin actually works. I said earlier that insulin is important to allow sugar into our cells. Without insulin sugar cannot get into our cells very well.

As an aside, when we are exercising our muscle cells allow sugar in with very little or no help from insulin. But how exactly does insulin help sugar get into our cells?

In order for insulin to allow sugar into our cells, it first binds to the outside part of the cell. This outside part is known as a cell membrane. When insulin binds to the cell membrane it sends a message to the inside of the cell. Insulin can do this because the place where insulin attaches to goes through the entire cell membrane and causes changes in the inside of the cell. The changes that occur are what allow sugar to finally get into the cell.

Since insulin is the first thing that carries the message, the message to let sugar in, it is called the first messenger. Once insulin attaches to the cell surface, it sends a signal through the cell membrane causing a release of chemicals called the second messengers. It is these second messengers that eventually let sugar into the cell and it is the overuse of these second messengers that gets us into trouble. How many people know that insulin causes cell damage in and off itself? We need to examine what, exactly, this second messenger does to give the cell the message to let sugar in.

Two things relay the second message. One is a substance called IP3 (inositol 1,4,5-triphosphate) and the other is

DAG (diacylglycerol). These two things come from the breakdown of something called phosphatidyl inositol 4,5-bisphosphate (also known as PIP2).[2] Now don't lose me; it really isn't difficult to follow through.

To recap, insulin binds to the outer part of the cell and is referred to as the first messenger. The attachment of insulin to the outer part of the cell sends a message to the inside of the cell. The message insulin brings is to break apart PIP2 into IP3 and DAG. It is IP3 and DAG which are the second messengers.

Now this doesn't seem like a big deal. Heck, we need to get sugar into the cell. We'd rather have it in the cell instead of outside the cell. In fact, if sugar stays outside the cell as I have mentioned before, it will start to attach to things it shouldn't, and will cause a malfunctioning of cells and then organs. This is what causes the side effects of diabetes, which we'll discuss in Part 2.

Anyway, in order to get the sugar into the cell, we need the help of IP3 and DAG. The problem is not with IP3. The problem lies with DAG. DAG stood for diacylglycerol, just

2   ibid, p.344-46

a fancy way of saying 2 acyls and a glycerol. It is with one of these acyl things that all havoc breaks lose.

Now, acyl is just a big fancy way of saying a long fat chain. So this diacylglycerol contains two long fat chains, as di means two. The problem is that one of these fat chains is something called arachidonate. Arichidonate is the starting point for the creation of extremely important signaling molecules. These are known as prostaglandins, prostacyclins, thromboxanes and leukotrienes.[3] The other term we use for these signaling molecules is eicosanoids. (An excellent review of this whole process can be found in Barry Sears, *The Zone*.)

In fact, an enzyme known as diacylglycerol lipase breaks down DAG into arachidonate. Then the signaling molecules, the eicosanoids, can be made. My physician readers will recognize most, if not all, of these signaling molecules.

The problem with these signaling molecules is that they may not send nice messages to our cells. The prostaglandins

---

3   Ibid, p. 624

are known to allow us to feel pain and to promote the development of clot formation by making platelets stickier. Thromboxanes have the opposite effect, they make platelets less sticky. The leukotrienes will allow us to experience a worsening of allergy symptoms, including asthma. Arachidonate has also been implicated in sending signals for tumor (cancer) growth as well as sending signals to allow cancer to spread (metastasize). If you want to scare yourself go to your favorite search engine and perform a search of arachidonic acid and cancer. How many hits did you get? It has been known for years that arachidonate sends cancer-promoting messages to our cell's DNA. Obviously not a good thing, but more about the cancer and carb connection later.

Let me put this all together. When we eat carbs our pancreas secretes insulin. Insulin allows us to make more cholesterol. Insulin also is anabolic in a sense that it prevents us from losing weight and helps us to gain weight. We also now know that insulin acts through a second messenger system. We also found out that one of these messengers, DAG, can be extremely dangerous. The more DAG, the more bad messages can be sent within our cells. The problem is that the more insulin we secrete, the more DAG is created. But it all goes back to what? Carbs. Carbs set into motion all of these bodily processes which are not good for us.

So it is essential we do not over eat carbs. What would be considered overeating? Well, if any of you have a medical problem requiring medication, you probably should not allow yourself anymore than sixty grams a day of carbs. If you're a diabetic, then no more than twenty or thirty at the most. Remember, it is absolutely imperative that before any of you start a low carb diet, you need to find an experienced low carb doc who can watch you like a hawk. Do not, I repeat, do not under any circumstances start a low carb diet without first consulting your doc. If your doc tells you that you should not start a low carb diet — find another doc who knows what they're talking about.

I know this has been a long chapter, but it is an important one because it shows how insulin is involved in creating some very bad things. Now don't get me wrong, insulin is needed in small quantities, without it, we die. But the amounts that a typical person secretes each day are extraordinarily high. And it all goes back to carbs. It was the consumption of carbs which caused the insulin to show up in the first place. A little bit of insulin, fine. But the amount of insulin most people squirt out, well, it encourages cholesterol production, allows us to get fatter, and from the discussion above, sends signals to allow us to experience more pain and can increase our development of cancer. And this is just the tip of the proverbial iceberg. We all need to be afraid of insulin; we need to be very, very afraid.

CHAPTER NINE-PARTIALLY
HYDROGENATED OILS

My six-year-old daughter understands the dangers inherent in partially hydrogenated oils. When we are at a restaurant she'll ask if what she is eating is low carb and will oftentimes ask the server, "Are there partially hydrogenated oils in this food?" Of course the servers have not a clue what my daughter is talking about, even though she is asking about the presence of the most dangerous fat out there. Partially hydrogenated oils are nothing more than a FAKE fat, created in laboratories for ease of use by food manufacturers. Partially hydrogenated oils are also known as trans fats. You know they're present when you review the ingredient list and see 'partially hydrogenated soybean oil or partially hydrogenated cottonseed oil', the two most common. By law now the ingredients must list the amount of trans fats. But don't get too complacent.

A lot of side packaging labels will have zero grams of trans fat, but when you read the ingredient list you will notice it contains partially hydrogenated soybean oil. Well, what's up with that? The reason the food industry can get away with this is that if there is less than half a gram per serving (0.5 grams or 500 milligrams), they are allowed, by law, to put zero.

Well, I'm sorry, but the presence of 500 milligrams is not zero, at least not in my book. No pun intended. And the other problem is that it only takes microscopic amounts to wreak havoc on our systems. So what exactly is it about a trans fat that makes it so dangerous?

Well, a trans fat is so named because of how the molecule looks. A trans fat contains what are known as double bonds. Think of a trailer attached to a car by a hitch. Usually there's only one hitch. Now pretend that for a particular trailer you need to have two hitches attached to the car. This is kind of what a double bond is. It just means that things are attached to each other with two attachments, rather than one.

If a molecule contains a double bond things can be attached above or diagonally opposite in relation to the double bond. Don't get too crazy trying to visualize this. Suffice it to say that when things are attached diagonally opposite to the double bond it is referred to as trans. When things are placed above the double bond it is called cis. It's just the words biochemists use to describe where things are located in relation to the double bond.

Now if we have a double bond in a fat where the attachment just happens to be diagonally opposite, it is called a trans fat. Trans fats are fake, they are artificially produced. Since these fats are fake and artificial our bodies do not know how to break these trans fats down. In fact, we do not have any way to break these fats down safely. Specifically, we do not have the proper enzymes to get rid of these fats. The only fats we can break down are the cis fats.

When our bodies attempt to break down trans fats we produce a thing known as a free radical. Go to your computer, pick your search engine, and put in free radicals and cancer, or free radicals and heart disease. How many hits did you get? I know, a lot.

Free radicals are scary. Very scary. They wreak havoc on our systems because they want to attach to everything they come across. When we eat anything that contains a trans fat we cannot break it down, and it just goes throughout our bodies causing damage. The damage is generally on our arterial walls. This is why there is now said to be a correlation between trans fats and heart disease, as well as cancer.

At the cellular level trans fats may act as signals for cells to turn cancerous. Remember, I am referring to very small amounts of trans fats, which may cause this damage. Even half a gram, which isn't a lot, may be enough to cause arterial wall damage and possibly turn on cancer genes.

As a side note, in New York City there is a new law which bans trans fats from being used in public restaurants. This is a major step in the right direction. Trans fats should be illegal. No one should have to worry about coming across this deadly FAKE fat.

Some organizations are still promoting margarine as a substitute for butter. Margarine is a trans fat. We now know from our discussion that butter is very good for us. We know that eating butter will raise our HDL and will help us lose weight, as long as we're not putting the butter on a loaf of bread.

Now enter margarine. A trans fat. I told you above what trans fats are and why they are deadly, not just dangerous. Why would any one in the world advertise margarine as safe? You got me. You now know better. So don't eat things with trans fats in them.

As another interesting side note I came across an e-mail about how plastic and margarine were only one molecule away from being the same. I did some research and found this to be not entirely accurate. Specifically, when making vinyl plastic, molecules of a substance known as ethylene are forced by heat to attach to one another. It appeared as if there were only single bonds present, not the trans bonds we talked about above. In reality margarine more closely resembles rubber. Rubber contains double bonds like margarine, although in a cis configuration, not trans. I'm not sure what causes me more concern, food resembling plastic, or foods related to rubber. You be the judge. The e-mail did mention that if you left margarine out in your backyard, no insects would touch it. I have not tried this experiment yet, but I will, and report back on my results later. I will not be surprised if no insects are found trying to 'eat' margarine, as margarine is devoid of any useful nutritive value for us humans as well. And I am picking on us doctors because some of us have promoted margarine as being safe, when it is not. Here it appears insects are smarter than us doctors.

CHAPTER TEN-NON-NUTRITIVE SWEETENERS

Non-nutritive sweeteners need to be mentioned because when we eat low carbs we will come across these things. The most widely seen are Nutrisweet (also known as aspartame), Stevia (a mixture of over a hundred herbs from something known as Asteracea now banned in the US, but can be found in other countries), Splenda (dextrose, maltodextrin, sucralose), Equal (dextrose, maltodextrin, aspartame), Sweet-n-Low and the like. They are referred to as non-nutritive because they provide a sweet, sugary taste to the foods we eat; yet they contain no nutrition such as carbs, protein, fat, vitamins or minerals. They may be placed in foods which have nutrients, but the sweetener itself is absent of any nutrition in and of itself. You will be bombarded with foods which contain, most commonly, the controversial aspartame. So what exactly is aspartame, and why the controversy?

Aspartame is formed when we combine an amino acid, phenylalanine, with another amino acid called aspartic acid.[1] This new substance is about 100 times as sweet as table sugar. Since it does not contain any carbs it will not put weight on you and it cannot be used to make cholesterol or fat.

The controversy is the anecdotal reports of aspartame being associated with everything from multiple sclerosis to Gulf War Syndrome. I have read numerous internet reports sent by concerned people speaking of all the dangers inherent in aspartame. The only problem is, there is no factual scientific evidence that aspartame causes any problems, unless you are born with a deficiency in a certain enzyme (phenylalanine hydroxylase) and cannot break down the phenylalanine part of aspartame. Thing is, in the US, we check for a deficiency of that enzyme at birth, so we should not be missing the absence of the enzyme unless the newborn isn't checked.

---

1   *Organic Chemistry*, Solomons & Fryhle, Seventh Edition, p.1122

But hold on, I told you that aspartame is a combination of both phenylalanine and aspartic acid; maybe it's the aspartic acid part causing the problems. Well, aspartic acid is also known as aspartate, which is simply an amino acid. Amino acids are the building blocks of protein. Without amino acids, proteins cannot be built. If proteins cannot be built in our bodies, we die. When we eat proteins our bodies break down the protein into what made up the protein in the first place, that is, the amino acids. So our bodies are used to seeing these amino acids and we need them to survive.

The Internet reports I read blamed the many diseases aspartame allegedly caused on the presence of formaldehyde. In other words, the concerned citizens were stating aspartame was somehow creating formaldehyde and it was the formaldehyde, which caused all the diseases.

Now while aspartame does break apart in solution, which limits its shelf life, and it is troublesome to cook with for the same reason; it does not break apart in any way to create formaldehyde. I suppose someone who had a little bit of chemical knowledge may have looked at the structure of aspartame and compared it to what formaldehyde looks like. The two at first glance look nothing like one another. But somebody wanted to find something wrong with aspartame so they continued to look.

Trouble is, the body does not break down aspartame in any way to form formaldehyde. It would take extreme heating in an attempt to create formaldehyde from aspartame and the heat it would take would cause everything to collapse into a bunch of single elements. Mainly carbon, hydrogen and oxygen. So, yeah, you'd get a lot of gas from the explosion you'd create to do this, but you would not make any formaldehyde. So basically even though there are look alike areas on aspartame that closely resemble formaldehyde, our bodies cannot and do not break down aspartame to create formaldehyde. Our bodies break up aspartame into phenylalanine and aspartate, two amino acids our body's can handle. I may have failed to mention that phenylalanine is also an amino acid, but it is, and it too, is safe.

Some, who have read of the dangers relating to aspartame, may remember the soda can scenario. It was argued that formaldehyde was produced in the soda cans in the Gulf War, due to the extreme heat of the desert. This seems logical until one realizes that the amount of heat needed to possibly create formaldehyde from aspartame would be so high, the cans would explode. Then of course, you wouldn't be able to drink the soda.

When one finally understands aspartame, one can see that it is safe to drink or eat. It is not a dangerous sweetener and I consume it on a daily basis and I haven't had an issue with it; and I've been eating and drinking products with aspartame for as long as I can remember. Actually, if you stop and think about it, aspartame is found in just about every diet product out there. Millions and millions of people ingest it every day. Why haven't we seen a statistically significant rise in all the diseases aspartame is reported to cause? Until I see some evidenced-based scientific data showing aspartame is dangerous, I'll continue to eat or drink it on a daily basis.

Aspartame is found in a sweetener known as Equal. We have already discussed aspartame, but now we need to discuss the other ingredients in Equal, that is, the dextrose and maltodextrin. I get a little anxious when I find dextrose and maltodextrin in an ingredient list. This is because dextrose is just a fancy way of saying glucose and maltodextrin is glucose molecules attached together, but not long enough to represent a true carbohydrate. In biochemistry speak, it is a short chain carbohydrate. Yes, both dextrose and maltodextrin have the potential to make cholesterol and fat, as well as elevate blood pressure and sugar numbers. I will tell my patients if they are having a hard time with lowering their cholesterols, losing weight, lowering blood pressure, or are still seeing elevated blood sugars to avoid Equal to see what effect that has. If things correct themselves, then they are told to stay off equal, if nothing happens then they are told they can continue with this sweetener.

As far as Splenda is concerned, it too, contains dextrose and maltodextrin so the same cautionary advice holds, but its last ingredient is a substance known as sucralose. Sucralose is claimed to be about 600 times as sweet as sucrose. (Ibid)

Sucrose is commonly known as table sugar and contains both glucose and fructose combined together. Sucralose is an artificial sweetener, will not cause tooth decay, and can be used in baking. (Ibid) Our bodies do not treat sucralose as it does sucrose. That is, sucralose will not be broken down into glucose and fructose, therefore no cholesterol, fat, blood pressure or sugar elevations should be seen with sucralose. Of course, if one sees elevations to the above, then one must stop their consumption of any foods which contain sucralose.

Now a word about saccharin. Yes, an experiment many years ago suggested saccharin caused cancer in lab rats. Problem is, they were giving these poor rats what would be equivalent to a few tons of the stuff for us, over a short period of time. Heck, even water can kill us if we drink too much of it. And then the scientists found out that a mite, which infected the rats, was creating the cancer. I do consume saccharin, not so much on a daily basis, but I am certainly not convinced it causes cancer.

How many of you know about the mite, saccharin, and cancer link? I'm thinking not many. Well, let's see, why did this not make it in the paper? Got me. All I can say is until you know the facts, you just don't know. Since I know the facts, I am not afraid to consume foods containing these sweeteners.

CHAPTER ELEVEN-MORE ON
CHOLESTEROL

At the risk of really boring you and I hope I haven't done so already, we need to talk a little bit more about cholesterol. To refresh, you know that our bodies make cholesterol from sugar, and we know there are many sugar molecules linked together in carbohydrates. We also know that whole grains and fruits, two of the most common food items touted as being healthy, contain enormous amounts of sugar.

I went through how eating cholesterol sends signals to the cell to stop making the enzymes necessary for cholesterol production. So we already know that eating cholesterol actually helps lower the production of cholesterol inside us. In fact, the only thing I've seen clinically raise HDL (the good cholesterol) has been the consumption of cholesterol. I do not know why this is the case, I only know it's true clinically. Just because I'm ignorant as to why eating more cholesterol raises your HDL doesn't mean it's not rue, or that it is wrong. So you docs out there be careful about saying I'm crazy because what I've seen clinically is a fact.

Now remember we talked about all those DLs, you know, the HDL and the LDL (we can ignore the IDL and VLDL for now). I talked a little bit about what these things were made up of. Let me add that inside these DLs are poly and monounsaturated fatty acids. These types of fatty acids are said to help lower one's risk for heart disease, that is, the poly and monounsaturated fatty acids.

What is a poly or monounsaturated fatty acid? I talked a little bit about double bonds above. Well, poly (which means many) and mono (which means one) simply means these are fatty acids that have either many double bonds or one double bond. That's it. Pretty simple.

Biochemically speaking, the more double bonds you have in a fat, the softer it is. Cooking oils are said to be healthy for you. They are mainly made up of polyunsaturated fatty acids (remember that you can use fatty acid and triglyceride interchangeably). What do you know about the consistency of cooking oil? That's right, it's an oily liquid.

Now butter contains saturated fats. Saturated fats are so named because they have no double bonds. As an aside, if a double bond exists, we have the potential to connect something to that bond. If no double bond exists, we cannot attach anything else to that bond. Therefore, we use the term saturated. Kind of like when your whole body is soaking wet with rain and there is not a part of your body that isn't wet, we refer to that as being saturated. Similar thing with saturated fats.

Saturated fats are supposed to be bad for us. The poly and monounsaturated fatty acids are supposed to be good for us. But why? I hate to admit it, but I am ignorant as to why poly and mono are ok and saturated is bad. I cannot find any scientific explanation as to why, just anecdotal information. I use anecdotal as meaning that somebody, usually a scientist or doc who's well respected, makes a statement about something and this statement is believed to be true without any further verification. Why should we not believe them, they know what they're talking about, right?

Well, I hate to be the naysayer, but they sometimes do not know what they're talking about. In my practice when I have my patients eat either saturated, mono or polyunsaturated fatty acids, they loose weight, their sugars normalize, their TGs lower and I see a lowering in blood pressures as well, among many other positive health benefits. I do not see a worsening of the lab reports when I check them. I haven't seen clinically that either fat is any worse or any better for you. To make matters even more interesting, HDL and LDL cholesterols both contain mono and polyunsaturated FAs.

That's right, the LDL, which we learned to be skeptical of as it's a calculated value, actually contains mono and polyunsaturated FAs. So if I'm lead to believe that mono and polyunsaturated FAs are good for you, but LDL is bad for you, how do I reconcile this with the fact that the 'bad' LDL contains the 'good' fatty acids? Could it be that the 'powers to be' got it wrong? That would be the only explanation if

LDL were actually bad for you. We now know the HDL and LDL molecules are much more complicated than once thought. Now enter the VAP test.

VAP stands for Vertical Auto Profile test. It is a newer way to check the actual DLs in our blood and is a better predictor of possible future heart problems. The VAP test is based on the fact that the HDL and LDL molecules actually consist of sub molecules. In other words, there are different HDL molecules and different LDL molecules. In fact, for LDL, there is good LDL and bad LDL, and for HDL, there also exists good and bad HDLs.

Talk about confusing. We can have high levels of bad 'good' cholesterol and low levels of good 'bad' cholesterol; or, preferably, low levels of bad 'good' cholesterol, high levels of good, 'good' cholesterol, low levels of bad, 'bad' cholesterol and high levels of good 'bad' cholesterol.

Have a headache yet. Definitely confusing, but a darn good test to help identify, as far as what we now know, more precisely what's going on with the DLs in your blood. If your doc does not order the VAP test, ask for it. It will take them a little more time to interpret it, but it will provide better guidance as to whether or not your profile needs improving. The VAP test is especially important if you have a high total cholesterol and a high HDL. It will allow us to actually measure whether the HDL is indeed the 'good' HDL and will show us whether the LDL is truly 'bad'.

OK, enough about cholesterol, let's talk about the food pyramid.

CHAPTER TWELVE-THE FOOD PYRAMID

My description of the food pyramid only requires one word—WRONG! The food pyramid is a representation of how we shouldn't be eating if we want to stay healthy. It allows for way too many carbs, and does not allow enough for protein, fat or cholesterol.

We already learned that eating fat would not make us fat, as long as we are not eating too many carbs. We also learned the major contributor to our cholesterol number is what our body produces, and we now know that our body produces this cholesterol from carbs. We also learned that the more cholesterol we eat, the less our bodies make. So why on earth would the food pyramid allow for the over consumption of carbs, and limit consumption of the very things our body needs to stay healthy. In one word, ignorance. Ignorance from the medical profession in regards to how we really should be eating. Ignorance of the well funded three letter organizations that, unfortunately, propagate ignorant dietary guidelines. Everything I have been stating about low carb diets is based on factual biochemical and clinical evidence and can only be refuted if one is, shall I say, ignorant.

The food pyramid should not be followed, unless, of course, you want to become a diabetic, gain weight, get high blood pressure, increase the dangerous cholesterol in your blood, raise your TGs, increase your risk of cancer and the list does not end there.

Time and again I walk into my examining room with recent lab work on a patient. The HDL is low and the TGs are through the roof. In case you're wondering, yes, this is a bad profile. Then I ask my patient how are they eating? The comment "Doc I'm eating a very healthy, well balanced diet."

"I see" I respond.

When I report the results of the lab work I'll often get the response "Well, I don't understand, I eat low fat and I rarely eat cholesterol, so I don't understand how my numbers can be so bad."This is when I start to explain how carbs are the culprit and how eating fat and cholesterol are actually safe. I sometimes get a weird look, like I'm crazy, but I persevere. I tell them that their 'well-balanced diet' is actually balanced in favor of carbs, and contains very little, if any, fat, protein or cholesterol

I always cringe when my patient's say they are eating a well balanced, healthy diet, because I know darn well it is going to be loaded top heavy with carbs. But it isn't my patient's fault. They have been brain washed into thinking how they're eating is ok. This is reflected in the food pyramid and almost the entire dietary information one comes across through magazines, books (not mine, of course), radio, TV, their doctor's offices and the like. As I mentioned earlier we are born and raised being indoctrinated what to believe as far as diet is concerned. Let me stress that again, we are indoctrinated with *what to believe* is the right way to eat.

But how to eat should not be based on what anyone believes and tells us, no matter how many degrees they have or what department of medicine they are in charge of. It should be based on scientific and clinical facts. We have accepted a low fat, low cholesterol diet, even though there is no scientific data or clinical evidence to support it. We arrived at that diet through a priori reasoning, told to us by people who were incorrectly educated in dietary sciences, then proposed an idea, and then held tenaciously on to that idea, no matter how often, clinically, that idea was disproved.

I must mention that I really only began low carbs after I proved to myself the biochemistry was real. I first put myself on low carbs, ate more fat, cholesterol and protein, and within six months was off the medications I was taking. I would like to repeat something worth repeating; DO NOT STOP ANY MEDICATIONS without first consulting with a doc who knows and has used low carbs in practice.

I actually backed into the biochemical explanation *after* I started low carbs. Even though *Protein Power* gave a wonderful explanation of what low carb diets are and why they work, as a physician, I tend to be skeptical. Before I knew low carbs worked, I was too skeptical, not allowing myself to even consider the possibility that low carbs could be beneficial. *Protein Power* opened my eyes because I immediately understood the biochemistry was real. After low carbs worked for me, that's when I re-read all my cellular physiology and biochemical textbooks to see where I went wrong.

What I found out was the biochemistry was taught right; it was the conclusions based on the biochemistry which was wrong. This was because a prior reasoning was used, not the facts as depicted in the already delineated biochemical pathways, and there was no clinical evidence (at least that I knew of) out there to allow me to question any hypothesis. So I accepted as gospel what I was told. That is, until I woke up.

So again, do not follow the food pyramid's recommendations unless you want to be unhealthy. I am aware that a new food pyramid is being considered. I have seen an example of it and it is still wrong. The new pyramid still allows for too many carbs and not enough protein, fat or cholesterol.

This new pyramid is not being released for a few years yet.

Thank goodness, maybe by that time the rest of the medi-

cal profession will wake up; but I sincerely doubt it.

OK, so enough about the food pyramid for now, let's get

on to the next chapter.

CHAPTER THIRTEEN-ALCOHOL

Let's face it; a lot of us drink alcohol socially, and I am talking about the alcohol that's safe to drink, not methanol or rubbing alcohol. So it is important to say a word or two about alcoholic beverages and low carb diets.

There are generally three categories of alcohol; beer, wine and the hard liquors. Alcohol is an interesting critter as the body treats the alcohol as a carb. This could have a double whammy effect, in a sense if you're drinking wine or beer, there will be carbs present in addition to the alcohol. If one has a mixed drink, say, a vodka and orange juice, the alcohol in the vodka will be treated as a carb as well as the sugar in the orange juice. Thus, the body sees more 'carbs' than with either the vodka or orange juice alone.

As a general rule of thumb if you like beer, you don't have to stop, unless, of course you're an alcoholic and need to.

There are plenty of low carb beers out there. As a beer drinker, I've done some personal studies for you, in the name of science of course. The lowest carb containing beer I've come across is a beer called Accel, but I cannot find it anymore. I never actually tried it, but no matter, as it appears to have disappeared anyway. Next in line are Michelob Ultra and Aspen Edge, both of which contain 2.6 grams of carbs per 12 ounce serving. Miller Lite has 3.1 grams and Bud Select has 3.2 grams.

Other common beers like Coors Light and Corona Light both contain 5 grams of carbs per serving; while Bud Light contains about 6 grams of carbs per 12 ounces. Watch out for Michelob Light, as it has more carbs than Mich Ultra. Budweiser is around 10 grams of carbs. Unfortunately, dark beers like Bass Ale and Guinness don't list the carb amount, so I cannot comment on them, but I am thinking it's more than 10 grams. It is important to note that you must count the carbs in the beer along with any other foods you consume with a meal. If you don't, you will wind up with too many carbs and you know the rest.

Now I am not a wine drinker, but I'll share what I know. For dry whites and reds, it's about a gram of carb per ounce. When going with a port wine, watch out, because all I can say is it's loaded with carbohydrates. Wine, in general, is made from grapes of course, and tends to be loaded with sugar, so be very careful when drinking it on a low carb diet.

Hard liquors, which I don't imbibe, can have anywhere from zero grams of carbs (vodka), to having a lot. So if you drink it, make sure you check the carb content. And a final word to the wise, watch your intake. For guys, they say (I have no idea who 'they' are, I'll try to find out for you) no more than 3 drinks a day, be it 3 beers, 3 glasses of wine (I'm assuming 4 ounces per glass, but you know what happens when we assume), or 3 one-ounce hard liquor-containing drinks per day. For women, it's only 2 beers, 2 glasses of wine or 2 ounces hard liquor per drink.

I used to think this study was performed by a male (to let us guys drink more), but what I've seen clinically is that women tend to be more sensitive to the bad effects of alcohol. This is seen mainly in elevated liver enzymes, which signifies irritation to the liver. If the irritation persists, liver disease and possibly cirrhosis may develop. Cirrhosis is death to the liver, it cannot be reversed once it happens, and can kill you. So, again, be careful with the consumption of alcohol, especially those of you with diabetes and high blood pressure, which I'll talk more about later.

CHAPTER FOURTEEN-WHAT ABOUT ALL THOSE STUDIES *PROVING* LOW FAT/LOW CHOLESTEROL DIETS WORK?

This can be answered quite simply, they don't. I have never come across a low fat, low cholesterol study which showed as dramatic an improvement in TGs, HDLs or blood sugars, as compared to the low carb diet. It is interesting to note that when the powers that be allegedly study the effects of low carb diets on TGs, cholesterol or blood sugar, the result is almost always the same; the studies appear to show low carb diets do not work.

The reason the low carb diets appear not to work is because when the experimenter's perform the study, they allow for too many carbs, thus messing up any possible positive outcome. More carbs are allowed usually in the form of, guess what, fruits and whole grains. Fruits and whole grains are introduced into these allegedly low carb diet studies because the research people honestly feel these things are safe, or maybe they feel that these foods represent natural sugars and should not be regarded as dangerous. They just don't get that when fruits and whole grains are present all the signals are sent throughout our bodies to do the bad things I already mentioned. They do not understand that sugar is sugar is sugar. Heck, if you think about it, *all* sugar is natural.

That's right, all sugar is natural. Even the sugar in say, a snickers bar, or the crumb cake you love so much. Most of the sugar is either high fructose corn syrup, or some variant thereof. Well, where do you think the high fructose part comes from? That's right, fructose comes from fruit. Fruit is natural, isn't it? Now where do you think the corn syrup part is derived from? Hmmm, let's see, the phrase is *corn* syrup. We see corn mentioned, so maybe corn syrup comes from corn? Isn't corn considered natural too? So by very logical reasoning, and it is indeed true, high fructose corn syrup comes from fruit and corn, two, what I would consider, very natural things. I hate to blow a hole in anyone's bubble, but so-called natural sugar is just as dangerous and deadly. So please always remember, sugar is sugar is sugar and natural sugar is not safer.

So anytime you read or watch or hear that the low carb diets do not work, remember, it was not even a low carb study to begin with. This is absolutely frustrating to doctors like me who know that the study which incorrectly showed low carbs do not work, was performed incorrectly.

I said the results when low carb diets are studied almost always result in negative outcomes, but there have been true low carb studies done thanks to Dr. Robert Atkins. In one study he either funded or directed (or both), the low carb diet worked wonderfully to lower TGs, raise HDLs and lower blood sugar. These results were seen because an actual low carb diet was done and studied properly. Dr. Atkins was an absolute pioneer in the understanding and implementation of low carb diets and is someone I wished I had had the opportunity to meet.

Patients have often asked me since I care for thousands of people, why don't I just perform my own scientific study and put one group of patients on low carb and the other group on a low fat, low cholesterol diet? My response is always the same, "Why would I need to perform a study when I know what the clinical outcome will be, and knowing this, why would I want to place anyone on a low fat, low cholesterol diet?"

It's the same reason why when low carb diet studies are done, fruits and whole grains are introduced. It's because the researchers feel and believe that these things are safe and are probably afraid not to keep those things in the diet. But this is where they are wrong. I am not working on a belief system and I do not *feel* low carb diets are correct. The reason I use low carb diets in my practice is because I have seen them work. Not just in principle, but in practice.

Remember that if you eliminate all the cholesterol from your diet, you'll lower your cholesterol by about ten percent. For the low fat, low cholesterol proponents this will be viewed as a wonderful feat. But unfortunately, it is not enough to keep most of us off meds. It wasn't enough for me, even following the strictest of low fat, low cholesterol diets.

Another statement very commonly heard is that "we do not know the effects of staying on these low carb, high fat, high cholesterol and high protein diets, for long term." First off, we do know the long-term effects. The long term effects seen by me through my patients is that these patients stayed healthy, with little if any medical problems, on little, if any medications, as long as they were on the low carb diet.

Second off, while the diet I'm talking about here is low carb, it is *not* a high fat, high cholesterol or high protein diet. The other thing it is not is low carb, low fat, low cholesterol, and high protein. This is another common error patients make because that's what they think they hear from me in the examining room, when I am discussing diet. A good proportion of patients I have my lengthy talk with about the correct way to eat, still leave my examining room hearing low carb, low fat, low cholesterol, high protein. These patients are battling against the brainwashing of many years being told that low fat, low cholesterol dieting is the way to go. They just have mistakenly combined low fat, low cholesterol with low carbs. Of course this is immediately corrected and they get on the right track at a subsequent encounter with me.

I must also make a statement that it appears as if more physicians understand that some carbs, that is, the so-called 'white carbs' are bad for you (white bread, white pasta, and white rice), but these physicians still hold on tenaciously to the fallacy that fruits and whole grains are ok. Although these doctors are coming to the understanding that carbohydrates and simple sugars are bad for the patient; they need to take that next step and realize that all sugars are bad.

We learned earlier that sugar is sugar is sugar. There is no such thing as a good carb. This is because, and I cannot stress it enough, sugar is sugar is sugar. Again, it does not matter if the sugar molecule comes from a snickers bar or a piece of fruit. The body will do with this sugar molecule what the body will do with this sugar molecule; and that is, the body will make more fat, cholesterol, and increase your risk for all types of cancer. Period. And that's just the tip of the iceberg. There are no ifs, ands, or buts.

CHAPTER FIFTEEN-VEGETARIANISM

A vegetarian is someone who does not eat meat. There are your lacto vegetarians, those who don't eat meat or drink milk. And there are your lacto-ova vegetarians, those who don't eat meat, eggs or drink milk. For the most part a vegetarian diet consists of carbohydrates, unless one is eating a lot of soy. Soy is one way a vegetarian receives protein in their diet.

Vegetarian diets provide the body with all the signals to make more cholesterol, make and store more fat, and also sends the signals to our cells, which can result in cancer. And that is only the beginning. No, vegetarian diets are not safe, not at all.

Another problem with vegetarian diets is that they do not provide one with any Vitamin B 12. Vitamin B 12 comes only from animal sources. No vitamin B 12 is found in plants. But, vegetarians will argue, breads are enriched with B 12. Well, the problem with the whole enrichment process is that the amount of B 12 placed in, say, bread, is not even enough to help with the bread's own digestion. You see, B 12 is an important vitamin as it allows us to extract energy from foods. Without B 12 it is very difficult to get energy out of food and this is why a lot of vegetarians are fatigued.

Most vegetarians have told me that the reason they are vegetarians is because they believe (there goes that belief thing again) that a vegetarian lifestyle is healthier and they argue our digestive systems prefer plant food to animal food. Why else, goes the argument, do we have all these problems with high cholesterol and high fats in the blood? Using a priori reasoning it is easy to see how vegetarians arrived at this incorrect conclusion. Avoid the things that contain cholesterol and fat and your cholesterol and fat numbers should get better. Unfortunately for the vegetarian, this is not true, and it is wrong, dead wrong. With an emphasis on the dead.

One only has to compare our digestive tracks with a known carnivore, say, a wolf, with a known herbivore, say, a cow, to see why humans were never meant to be eating plants. A carnivore is an animal that eats meat, while an herbivore eats plants only. When we compare our digestive system with that of a wolf, we find it is very similar. When we compare our digestive system with a cow, there is no similarity whatsoever. Hmmm, so what do you think we should be eating?

CHAPTER SIXTEEN-KETOSIS

OK, so let's imagine that you've decided to start a low carb diet after reading some books on the topic. If you're not on any meds there's no reason why you cannot start immediately, although it's always better to start under the guidance of a doc experienced in low carb diets. So you may have read in some low carb books that you can tell if you're burning fat by checking the ketone levels in the urine.

Ketones are created when our body burns fat and these ketones will wind up in the urine. There are things called 'ketostix' on the market that actually measure the ketone level in the urine. Some of the books suggest you check your ketone levels so you know whether or not you're burning fat.

I usually recommend against checking ketone levels in the urine. If you are losing weight, you know you're burning fat, as long as you are eating enough protein and fat. There is no reason to check the ketones in the urine because they will be there. So save your money.

Sometimes doctors confuse benign dietary ketosis (BDK) with that of the life threatening diabetic ketoacidosis (DKA). DKA is found almost exclusively in Type I diabetics. Type I diabetics no longer make insulin. In fact, BDK is what some docs attempt to use to scare people into stopping low carb diets. True, DKA is life threatening and some of my patients have died because of DKA, but they were diabetics. I have never had a patient die or become ill because of BDK.

The docs who are using BDK as a scare tactic to get their patients to refrain from starting a low carb diet, do not understand BDK at all. If they did, they would not use BDK to frighten patients. This is another example of dietary ignorance.

Before I understood low carb diets, I too, used to use BDK as a scare tactic to frighten my patients. I would state that ketosis is a dangerous thing and could possibly cause death if it persists too long. I was confusing BDK with DKA, just like the bulk of docs who continue to do so today.

But if I had just stopped and thought about it, it would have been very clear to me that BDK and DKA are not the same. Not at all. The only thing they have in common is that both BDK and DKA have keto in them (benign dietary 'keto'sis and diabetic 'keto'acidosis). Yes, there are ketones present in both situations; but in BDK, there is no acidosis or elevated blood sugar.

Acidosis occurs when the pH of the body becomes acidic, that is, a lower pH is found. This acidotic state, as it is called, is created because sugar is not getting into the cells. Sugar is not getting into the cells because the pancreas is not producing enough insulin. In an attempt to survive our bodies use different methods to get energy. One way is to use fat for fuel, hence the ketones. Another way is to use muscle tissue for fuel. When muscle tissue is used for fuel a substance referred to as lactic acid is created and this helps to lower the pH into the acidic range. There are also other things that lower the pH (i.e., anaerobic metabolism), but the main point is that BDK is not associated with acidosis or elevated blood sugars.

Benign dietary ketosis is just that, benign. We do not have to worry about it. It has to happen in order for us to lose weight. I have heard some docs say that you can lose weight but there should never be any ketones in the urine. This is dietary ignorance at its finest. There is absolutely no way to lose fat without the creation of ketones, because ketones are the byproduct of fat digestion. If we are digesting and getting rid of fat, ketones will be created. End of story.

To those physicians out there who continue to tell their patients to lose weight, but keep the ketones out of the urine, please understand that is impossible to do. It's like telling your patients to jump in a lake naked, but don't get wet.

Is that possible?

CONCLUSION TO PART I

OK, well we have talked a lot about what happens in our bodies when we eat carbs. I've focused on the making of cholesterol, how we make fat from carbs, why we get fat from eating carbs and hinted a little bit about the connection between carbs and cancer. Now I want to look at actual medical diseases and how carbs and the avoidance of carbs influence these medical disease processes. This list will not be exhaustive and I'm still learning on a daily basis, but what I am about to reveal to you is quite shocking. Please keep in mind as you read Part 2 that I will mention a disease only if I have seen a positive clinical outcome, which more likely than not, was the result of lowering one's carbs.

Now, on to Part 2.

PART II-CLINICAL APPLICATIONS

Welcome to Part II. I used the term 'Clinical Applications' as I will discuss specific medical conditions that responded positively, to a low carb, more fat, more cholesterol, more protein regimen.

CHAPTER SEVENTEEN-POLYCYSTIC OVARIAN SYNDROME (PCOS)

I'll start Part II with polycystic ovarian syndrome. Since I will be arguing that how we are fed in the womb sets us up for what medical problems we are going to have before and after we're born, it seems appropriate to start our discussion with one of the most common reasons women have difficulty getting pregnant in the first place.

Polycystic ovarian syndrome (PCOS), as the name suggests, is a condition where there are many cysts in a woman's ovary. (Poly means many; cystic means cyst and ovarian means ovary.) Along with the multiple cysts in the ovary is the overproduction of substances called androgens. Androgens are male sex hormones and their presence makes it more difficult for women to get pregnant. Women with PCOS also have irregular periods and do not ovulate regularly, both of which make it more difficult to get pregnant. Another interesting fact about polycystic ovarian syndrome is that it is also associated with increased insulin levels in the bloodstream. It was the fact that PCOS was associated with high insulin levels that got me thinking low carb diets could help women with PCOS.

We have already discussed what causes increased insulin levels to appear in the bloodstream. Insulin levels increase when our pancreases see more sugar. So an immediate connection should be apparent. Perhaps we can treat PCOS by lowering the amount of carbs a woman eats per day.

As a family physician, I have had the opportunity to test this theory on a number of women unfortunate enough to suffer from PCOS. What these women had in common was the fact they were overweight, could not get pregnant, had hair growth where it wasn't wanted, some had deeper voices and they all had elevated insulin levels in the bloodstream.

When these women were placed on a low carb diet, and followed it, some very interesting things began to happen. For starters, they began to lose the hair growth where it wasn't wanted, their voices became more feminine, and they started to lose weight. When insulin levels were checked three months after starting a low carb, more fat, more cholesterol, more protein diet, the insulin levels were lower.

What was even more fascinating is that when ultrasounds were done to actually visualize the cysts in the ovaries, the cysts began to disappear. Some women who remained on a low carb diet for six months had complete resolution of the cysts within their ovaries.

I have had women who could not conceive, even some who underwent infertility treatments, get pregnant after being on a low carb diet for about a year. I have seen this frequently enough to question the rationale of the use of infertility treatments on women with PCOS. It seems clear to me that before infertility treatments begin, dietary intervention should be tried first.

Of course the problem with dietary intervention is that it takes time to explain this to a patient in the examining room, and most docs don't want to 'waste their time' discussing this with their patients. This is because most people do not adhere to diets, and unfortunately the docs are correct in this regard. So it's easier to discuss what medical treatment options are available for infertility, as it's easier to offer a pill. Remember, us docs went to medical school to learn how to use medications to solve medical problems, we were not trained how to use diet to solve a medical issue.

I must stress that the success I've seen with women getting pregnant after starting low carb diets, has been in association with PCOS. And also remember that PCOS is a very common condition. Not all women with PCOS who started low carb diets became pregnant, but enough did that I make it a point when I meet a woman with PCOS, to have her start low carbs immediately. I continue this approach and see pregnant women routinely, some sent to me by their OB/GYN doc, for help in the treatment of PCOS. Changing the diet is definitely worth a try before starting medication.

As a side note, some OB/GYNs will use a medication called metformin to help with PCOS. Metformin helps by lowering insulin levels and this does help treat PCOS. I do not have much of an issue with this approach, but the metformin must be used in conjunction with a low carb diet. Using both metformin and a low carb diet will result in quicker resolution of the PCOS.

My final statement for this chapter will be if you are a woman who has difficulty conceiving and has been diagnosed with PCOS, you must start a low carb diet now. This is the only way to effectively treat PCOS. And of course you need to start low carbs with a doctor experienced in low carb diets.

CHAPTER EIGHTEEN–PREGNANCY

All I can say before I begin this chapter is grab a low carb snack and enjoy the discussion. This one is going to be an eye opener.

So let's start by assuming, and we all know what happens when we assume, your doctor was smart enough to have you start low carbs once you were diagnosed with PCOS. Both you and your doctor were amazed when the PCOS disappeared after you started low carbs, and guess what, the pregnancy test was positive. You are very excited. You cannot believe you are pregnant because you went through three infertility treatments without getting pregnant. But now you are. You ask yourself, "Was it really the low carb diet?" You're not sure, but no matter because you're pregnant and that's all that counts.

I have seen this happen often enough to know it was the low carb diet. The most common response of the

OB/GYN doc is to comment, "You were going to get pregnant anyway." Most OB/GYNs usually ignore the low carb diet as having had any influence on the pregnancy. My problem with this is that I have seen too many women have too many infertility treatments, which cost ten to twenty thousand dollars a treatment, all of which fail to result in a pregnancy; with the same women getting pregnant and delivering a very healthy baby, *after* starting a low carb diet, and *not* having had another infertility treatment. Hmmmm, interesting.

Now if you were on a low carb diet before pregnancy, the first thing your OB/GYN doc will tell you is to stop the low carb diet once you become pregnant. The reason is that everyone *knows* low carb diets are dangerous during pregnancy, right? Well, wrong again. Not only are low carb diets safe in pregnancy, but also for many women they are preferred.

I routinely place my diabetic, obese, and high blood pressure patients who become pregnant on a low carb diet. I must emphasize that they are placed on a low carb, more protein, more fat and more cholesterol diet. These patients do just fine remaining on a low carb diet throughout the pregnancy and deliver healthy babies at term.

Let's look at my gestational diabetic patients first. I will devote another chapter to diabetes but we need to examine diabetes in pregnancy and how it affects the developing baby. A woman who develops diabetes in pregnancy is said to have gestational diabetes. These women will have high blood sugars and also tend to be overweight. Sometimes the weight is gained during the pregnancy, but most of the time the woman goes into the pregnancy already overweight.

One of the most common complicaions of gestational diabetes is the so-called macrosomic infant. Macrosomic simply means big baby. Macro means large and somic means body, thus macrosomic means large body. This occurs because of the elevated blood sugar in the pregnant mom's bloodstream. The problem with a macrosomic baby is that the baby may not be able to fit through the birth canal. If this happens a caesarean section may need to be performed, with all the attendant risks of that surgical procedure, including the prolonged recuperative time which may interfere with maternal/newborn bonding.

Well it is true that the elevated blood sugar will create a baby that is large. So in an attempt to lower the blood sugar what do doctors suggest? We tell you to check your blood sugar and watch your diet. Doesn't sound too bad, but here's the problem.

First off, if your sugars are too high we will recommend that you avoid sweets, but will allow you to continue to eat fruits and complex carbs (whole grains). The thinking is that fruit is a natural sugar and complex carbs, because they are 'complex', will not elevate the blood sugar. Both of these assumptions are wrong. Fruit and complex carbo-hydrates will certainly elevate the blood sugar. After reading through this much of the book, we know this already. And if you remember that sugar is sugar is sugar, you will not fall into that trap anyway.

Well here's where the dietary ignorance of your doctor comes in. The first was thinking that fruit and complex carbs were safer, when they are not. By the way, a complex carb is a carb with millions of sugar molecules in it, just waiting to be set free. So when we eat a complex carb, the blood sugar stays higher for longer. Oopps. The second dietarily ignorant thing is in telling the pregnant mom to check her blood sugar a few hours *after* eating to see if the blood sugar is elevated. This is because when the blood sugar becomes elevated the sugar will pass through the placentae and create dangerous changes in the developing baby's physiology; by the time the pregnant mom knows the blood sugar is elevated, the damage has already been done. We'll discuss more about this later.

I disagree with the consumption of fruit and whole grains in an attempt to lower blood sugar. I disagree because it doesn't work. Never has, never will. I do not disagree with checking the blood sugar after eating, but I do disagree with the advice given if the blood sugar remains elevated. Now what do you think your doc is going to tell you to do if the blood sugar remains elevated? They're going to tell you it's not safe to have an elevated blood sugar and that the sugar needs to be lowered to prevent the baby from getting too big in the womb. This is all true. Well how do you think they are going to lower the blood sugar? It can't be diet because they already tried that and it didn't work. Remember, that was the fruit and whole grain thing. Your doc is now going to suggest you go on insulin to help lower the blood sugar and this is where your doc's dietary ignorance goes into supernova. A supernova is when a star explodes releasing billions of years of energy, created by a process called fusion, into the universe. This creates an explosion billions of times stronger than an atom bomb. No, this is not a compliment to us docs.

Now remember, I am not an OB/GYN, just a family doc who likes to think every now and then, and has a lot of experience in the field of OB/GYN. And I will admit I've made the same mistakes most of my colleagues are continuing to make. What makes me different is that I have made a conscious effort to be, shall I say, conscious. That is, I have started to think about some of the things us docs do, and take for granted, to see if they even make sense.

Unfortunately when it comes to treating a gestational diabetic, what we are trained to tell our patients is wrong. Very wrong. And armed with these ignorant dietary beliefs, doctors have the potential to kill not only a baby, but the mom as well.

So how exactly does the elevated blood sugar in the mom cause the baby to get bigger? Through insulin, and here's how. Every time the mom eats sugar, the sugar will pass through the placenta and wind up in the baby's bloodstream. When the baby's blood sees this sugar, the baby's pancreas will secrete insulin, just like ours. By the way, a baby can start to produce insulin at a very young developmental age, around ten weeks, maybe younger as newer studies are showing.

When the developing baby's pancreas squirts out insulin, it is the presence of the insulin in the bloodstream that causes the developing baby to get bigger. The more insulin a developing baby secretes, the bigger the baby gets. It's that simple. Remember that insulin is an anabolic hormone, which means insulin helps to make things bigger, and this is exactly what insulin is doing when a developing baby's pancreas secretes insulin.

In the chapter on obesity, I will explain the direct link between obesity and insulin. It is actually insulin that causes one to become obese through insulin's anabolic role, as we have talked about before.

OK, so why is this a testament to the dietary ignorance of physicians? Aren't doctors trying to help our gestational diabetic moms, and shouldn't that be enough? Well, the problem is that the doctors who are caring for these gestational diabetic moms are not thinking it through and that's where the ignorance plays in.

So we have a mom who is having high blood sugar in response to the eating of carbs. The doctor knows this because at about twenty eight weeks a test known as a glucola test is performed. This is a test where the pregnant mom drinks about fifty grams of sugar and the blood sugar is checked before and at specific times after drinking the sugar. By the way, a regular coke has approximately forty-four grams of sugar per twelve ounce serving, so this test is almost like having the soon-to-be mom drink a regular soda.

OK, so the mom comes in at twenty-eight weeks for this sugar test, drinks all this sugar, and then her doctor finds an elevated blood sugar. The problem is that no expecting mom should ever drink that much sugar in one sitting. A better way to test to see if blood sugars are elevated is to have the expecting moms check their blood sugars for a week, eating all the things they normally eat. If one finds an elevated blood sugar then the mom can be counseled as to what to eat, but they need to be counseled the right way.

When the pregnant moms drink all that sugar, what do you think happens? Yes, all that sugar eventually crosses through the placenta and makes its way into the new baby's blood. This will tell the baby's pancreas to secrete insulin and this will cause the baby to get bigger.

Now I know the OB/GYN's will argue that just one test with sugar, that is, the glucola test, should not cause a baby to get bigger, and I will agree. But the advice a pregnant patient gets after their sugar is found elevated is all-wrong.

We already know they are told to eat more fruit and whole grains, and we know this is wrong. When this doesn't work, the soon-to-be-moms are then told to check their sugar a few hours after eating carbs, and if the sugar is still elevated, to take an insulin injection. The insulin shot will help lower the blood sugar of the mom, but not the baby. This is because insulin does not cross the placentae.

Now here's where a doctor's dietary ignorance plays a part. First, if the expecting moms were told the correct way to eat, that is, to limit their carb intake, and to eat more fat, more cholesterol and more protein; their sugars would be normal and there would be no reason to have to take insulin at all. Second, checking the blood sugar a few hours after eating too many carbs allows sugar to pass into the developing baby's bloodstream. By the time the elevated blood sugar is found by the expecting mom, the sugar has already been in the baby's bloodstream a few hours. The baby's pancreas has already secreted insulin, and the baby's insulin has already sent all the signals needed for the baby to get bigger. All this happens *before the expecting moms even know their sugars are elevated.* Injecting insulin at this point only lowers the mom's blood sugar; and at this point, even if they are injecting insulin there is nothing they can do to prevent the sugar from having already been passed to the baby's bloodstream.

Explaining to an expectant mom the dangers of carbs will dramatically lower, if not eradicate, gestational diabetes. Please note, I am not referring to Type I diabetics who need to remain on their insulin throughout pregnancy. But even a Type I diabetic can prevent macrosomia by avoiding carbs. This is because even the blood sugar of a diabetic requiring insulin will remain better controlled on low carbs. Better control of blood sugar, less sugar makes it into the baby's circulation. Less sugar in the baby's circulation, less insulin secreted by our baby's pancreas. Less insulin secreted by the baby's pancreas, no more bigger babies. Problem solved. But the problem will not be solved until physicians realize their dietary ignorance and start telling our expectant moms the right way to eat. I hope this happens soon.

Another condition of pregnancy which is quite common and that low carbs will help, is that of pregnancy-induced hypertension (PIH). I have had many patients see me and they are scared to get pregnant because last time they were pregnant, their blood pressures were elevated. During that pregnancy they needed medications to help lower their blood pressures, and their docs were worried about two other related conditions, pre-eclampsia and eclampsia.

PIH is easy to treat once low carbs are started. I have used the low carb approach many times in women who had PIH, with wonderful and dramatic results. The problem with PIH is that when a woman presents with elevated blood pressure in pregnancy, they are immediately told to start a low fat, low cholesterol diet and to eat more whole grains and fruits. This is wrong. The only thing that dietary approach will succeed in doing is to elevate the blood pressure even further. If that dietary approach is followed, the women almost always need medications to control their BP, and now you have a pregnant woman on medications that their developing baby will now be exposed to. Not good.

I will discuss high blood pressure in a later chapter, but let me take the time to explain a little bit about high blood pressure now. High blood pressure is just that, it's elevated blood pressure in our arteries, capillaries and veins. This is bad because it causes a wear and tear effect on our arteries and over time can lead to heart attacks, strokes, vision problems, and kidney failure, just to name a few. In a pregnant woman it is a problem because blood pressures can become a little elevated in pregnancy, just because of being pregnant. So if you start off with elevated blood pressure and then get pregnant, your blood pressure can get even more elevated during the pregnancy. This is because there are a lot of fluid shifts going on when one is pregnant and this may lead to problems with blood pressure. Add swelling in the woman's ankles and protein in the urine along with the elevated blood pressure, and now you have a condition called pre-eclampsia.

High blood pressure is absolutely influenced by how many carbs one eats. The carbs will cause the pancreas to secrete insulin and two things we haven't discussed will happen.

First, the insulin will act within the kidneys and cause us to retain more salt, regardless of how much salt one is eating. More salt retention means, guess what, higher blood pressure.

Another thing that happens is that insulin will cause the smooth muscle cells of the arteries, and smaller arteries known as arterioles, which contain smooth muscle as well, to enlarge. When these smooth muscle cells enlarge, they narrow the diameter of the arteries and arterioles. Narrow the diameter of anything that carries fluid and the pressure will increase.

This is why lowering the carb content helps to lower blood pressure and the effect is dramatic in a pregnant woman. Lower the carbs in a woman with PIH and you normalize the blood pressure. And not only do you protect the pregnant woman, but you protect the baby as well. Normalizing the blood pressure in women with PIH will also prevent pre-eclampsia from even being seen.

It is important to note that eliminating pre-eclampsia from the equation means you'll never see eclampsia, the devastating, and life threatening clinical presentation of seizures during delivery. Eclampsia can take the lives of not only the pregnant mom, but their babies as well. All this can be prevented, from simply lowering one's carbs.

But what about a woman who is already pregnant and is overweight or obese, can she start low carbs *after* she is pregnant? Absolutely. Let me explain why.

That a pregnant woman should not lose weight, is another area of dietary ignorance doctors face. The thinking is that if the pregnant patient loses weight, this could affect the development of the baby. This is true and not true. It all depends on how the woman goes about trying to lose the weight. It is interesting to note that a lot of docs may object to my statement and say they encourage their overweight pregnant patients to lose weight, but few women are successful, because the guidance these women get from their docs is wrong. What do you think their docs tell them to do? That's right, eat more fruits and whole grains and that'll do the trick, that'll help you lose weight. Unfortunately we now know this is not true.

I have not answered the question why it is safe for a woman to start a low carb diet while pregnant. First, remember that we are talking low carb, more fat, more cholesterol, and more protein. *Not* zero carbs or *high* fat, *high* cholesterol or *high* protein. This needs to be repeated again and again and again, because over the years after having extensive discussions with thousands of patients, many leave the office thinking I said *no* carb, *low* fat, *low* cholesterol and *high* protein. This is exactly what I DID NOT SAY TO DO!

So let's get back to pregnancy. If you are already overweight going into a pregnancy, or if you are not over weight but did have problems with gestational diabetes, PIH, eclampsia, or pre-eclampsia in a prior pregnancy; if you do not watch your carbs with this new pregnancy, you are almost guaranteed to have the same problems you had with the last pregnancy.

I tell my pregnant patients to lower their carbs, just like I tell all my other patients who suffer from the diseases I have or will mention to lower their carbs. What I see clinically in my pregnant patients who are overweight or obese and lower their carbs, is that these patients lose weight during the pregnancy. Not only do these patients lose weight and continue to lose weight throughout the pregnancy, they give birth to very healthy babies whose weight is around 6–7 pounds. I have never seen a macrosomic baby delivered to a woman under my care who was following a low carb diet, never. And I never will. Remember, these women are eating lower carbs, but they are still eating what a developing baby needs, that is, protein, fat and cholesterol, and they are drinking plenty of fluids.

As a side note, if you look at what our bodies are made up of, we consist of the following; mainly water, depending on what book you read, some say as high as seventy percent water, with the rest of what we are made up of split between fat and protein. Carbohydrates make up only two percent of our bodies. A mere two percent. That's it. Yet, most diets out there allow for at least forty percent of the diet in the form of carbs. The majority of the diets unfortunately allow for about eighty percent of the foods to be carb-containing foods, with the remaining twenty percent split between protein and fat. This is wrong. Dead wrong.

Let's recap a bit. We have spoken about how a pregnant woman will do quite well if she maintains a low carb diet during pregnancy. Lowering the carbs can alleviate the need for any type of medical intervention for both the gestational diabetic and the patient with PIH. In addition, an obese pregnant patient who will almost surely give birth to a macrosomic baby, can give birth to a normal sized infant *and* remain healthy while losing weight throughout the pregnancy, if she stays on a low carb diet. All of these positive effects have to do with the lowering of insulin levels, which comes about when the women lower their carb intake.

I cannot say it enough, lower the carb intake and the insulin levels will lower. Since it was insulin causing all the problems in the first place, things like gestational diabetes, PIH and obesity in pregnancy can all be treated successfully, without meds, during pregnancy. Of course it behooves a woman who is thinking of getting pregnant to start low carbs as well.

I want to take time to discuss some things that I have been considering, that I believe may be contributing to the obesity and diabetes epidemic in our country and world-wide. I know I stated at the outset that I would only discuss things if I have personally seen it happen in my office, but I do have some ideas I know are important to share. Let me state quite forthrightly that I may be wrong, and would welcome any evidence to disprove my theory.

I have already mentioned a bunch of times that the pancreas squirts out insulin in response to carbohydrates. What I did not mention is that the pancreas retains a memory, for want of a better word, as to how much insulin it had secreted in the past. If the pancreas is always seeing a large amount of carbs, it will continue to secrete larger amounts of insulin than are actually needed. My question is this; could the embryological pancreas, due to very early exposure to large amounts of carbs, be pre-programmed to continually secrete larger amounts of insulin than are actually needed, throughout the pancreas's lifetime? Could the embryological pancreas be primed in utero (in utero refers to the developing baby while it is in the uterus), to always secrete more insulin, even when one eats lower carbs? Yes, it is supposition, but if it's true, we have an answer to the obesity and diabetes epidemic. A newborn's, child's, adolescent's and adult's pancreas, may actually be pre-programmed in-utero to secrete large amounts of insulin; and may continue to do so for the entire life of the individual.

Why is this the answer to the obesity and diabetic epidemic, because it is the insulin in our bloodstreams that makes us overweight and obese, with the subsequent development of diabetes. If the pancreas is not secreting large amounts of insulin, obesity and diabetes are curtailed. Remember also that insulin is responsible for both TG and cholesterol production. If we lower the exposure of the developing embryological pancreas to carbs, can we prevent a pre-programming and thereby allow the pancreas to secrete only the amount of insulin it needs to?

As an extremely interesting side note, I was born a macrosomic baby. I was about eight pounds thirteen and a half ounces at birth. Oh yeah, and my mom smoked while she was pregnant with me. Since smoking is known to cause lower birth-weight babies, could you imagine what my weight would have been if she didn't smoke? I suffered from obesity as a child and my mom had to starve me to help me lose weight. During medical school, I put on so much weight I tipped the scales at two hundred thirty two pounds. At only five foot six, I was obese. My blood pressure was high, my cholesterol profile stunk, and my sugars began to climb into the diabetic range.

I do not want to bore you with this story again, as I mentioned it in the preface, which nobody ever reads, so go back and read it, but I often wonder; was I set up to be obese, suffer from high blood pressure and have a bad cholesterol profile, even during my embryological and fetal development? I would say yes at this time, unless someone can offer me proof otherwise.

Getting back to the possible pre-programming of the pancreas, it is important to note that I am not talking about

Lamarkian inheritance, for those of you out there who may think that. Lamarkian inheritance is a belief in the inheritance of acquired characteristics. For example, if I work out all the time and develop big biceps, Lamarkian's believed that my son would be born with big biceps. There is a great book called, *The Case of the Midwife Toad*, I forget the author, but it's a wonderful read. This book examines our fascination with Lamarkian inheritance and how a scientist actually fudged data to try to prove this type of inheritance existed. The scientist was later found out to be a fraud. No, Lamarkian inheritance does not exist, nor am I suggesting that it does.

I ask this pre-programming question, as far as insulin secretion and the pancreas is concerned, because if the pancreas becomes pre-programmed to do this, this may set up a secretory pattern of the pancreas putting out too much insulin for each carb load it sees. Since we know that insulin is responsible, through its anabolic role, for obesity, as well as PIH, and it does have a role in the gestational diabetic; the more insulin the pancreas secretes, the more medical problems we see. Do not forget that it is also insulin that causes the majority of the macrosomic, or bigger babies out there, and that the lower the insulin level in the developing baby's blood, the less chance of having a bigger baby.

So it all goes back to insulin.

Insulin, insulin, insulin.

So what can we do to lower insulin levels?

Lower the carb intake.

Again, the pregnant mom who's watching her carbs will not only affect a positive change on *her* medical outcomes, but her developing baby as well.

So we now know it's important for moms to watch their carbs before and during pregnancy, but what about after pregnancy, the so-called post partum phase? Is it safe for a mom who is breastfeeding their baby to be eating low carbs? Well, what do you think my answer is going to be? That's right, of course it is! Good answer!

I am going to take time out right now and provide a brief public service message about breast-feeding. This message is being given for all those babies out there who are being breastfeed (thank goodness), to those mom's who can still begin to breastfeed, and to those moms who are wondering if they should breast feed.

I first start off my conversation with expectant moms who ask about breastfeeding by stating the following; "Women have two breasts, milk comes out of them, why do you think?" This may appear a bit harsh, but I think I make my point most of the time. There is nothing, absolutely nothing that compares to breast milk. No formula on the market even comes close to supplying the benefits of breast milk. Unfortunately, with witty advertising gimmicks and slogans, many parents are lulled into a false sense of complacency about formula, and think formulas provide almost an equal amount of nutrients.

I repeat again;

Formulas do not even come close to supplying a developing baby what is needed for their continued growth.

It is interesting that I did not even think much about breastfeeding and its importance until after I became involved with low carb diets. Sure, I received the rudimentary, oftentimes incorrect information in medical school and residency about breast-feeding. Remember the subtitle of my book, I was not, and still am not immune to being ignorant.

But the "Eureka!" bulb as to breast-feeding's importance did not go off, until I began to understand the importance of low crabs. (I mean carbs, not crabs. Although crabs are actually low carb, so they are ok to eat. I wonder how many times throughout this book I wrote crabs instead of carbs. So if you see low crabs, I really meant to say low carbs.) The importance of breast feeding becomes even clearer when one realizes that fat and cholesterol consumption is ok, and that breast milk contains a good amount of fat and cholesterol. Sure, breast milk does contain a good amount of carbs, and this is an argument I sometimes get, but breast milk also contains a large amount of cholesterol and fat, two things many of us are raised afraid to death to eat. Why do the low fat/low cholesterol proponents never bring up the fact that breast milk contains a large amount of fat and cholesterol? Got me. But like most people, and doctors are not immune to this, we only point to the evidence if it supports our claim. Mark Twain had a saying that "scientists use statistics like a drunkard uses a lamppost, generally for support, not for illumination?" I'll be the first to say I will gladly use data if it supports what I am saying, but I will also analyze contradictory data, and ask why I did not get the results I expected.

The problem is, for my critics, I can usually in a few seconds refute a claim or find a flaw in any study which thinks it proves low carb diets are dangerous, or that low fat/low cholesterol dieting is the way to go. Are any clinicians up to my challenge? I know a lot of you think you are, but I will advise you now, be very, very, careful. And make sure you know your biochemical pathways inside and out, because you'll need to know them.

Ok, back to breast-feeding. My final comment for pregnant women is to breast feed. If you have any questions refrain from asking your doctor before you talk to a lactation consultant, such as a La Leche counselor, as the advice most docs give on breast-feeding is wrong. Get answers first from the trained lactation specialist and then ask your doctor. Any answer you get from your doctor, think about critically. If there exists a large discrepancy in what the lactation consultant says versus your doc, get a second opinion from another doc.

Phew. Sorry it took me so long to get through this chapter. The problem is that pregnancy is so important and I have a lot to say about it. Believe it or not I can say a lot more, and I will.

Let's talk now about one of the major health epidemics facing Americans today.

Anyone care to guess?

That's right, it's obesity.

CHAPTER NINETEEN-OBESITY

We are fat in America. Really fat. And we continue to get fatter. Before you get insulted that I'm calling America fat, ask yourself;

Are you?

I was.

With the emphasis on 'was.'

Well if you are overweight, you are not alone. Instead of being insulted by my comments, and, by the way, I was considered morbidly obese at one time, understand that the reason you are overweight is most likely not your own fault. More likely the reason you are overweight, or possibly obese, is because of the dietary ignorance of physicians. The solution to America's obesity epidemic is out there, but most doctors are ignorant as to the reason behind why America is getting fatter. If you don't believe me that most doctors are dietarily ignorant about the obesity epidemic, just stop and point to all those fat doctors out there. There are a lot of them, heck, I was one of them.

Now what do you think I'm going to say is the reason for the obesity problem in our nation. It's a single word answer and it starts with I. It has three syllables.

Yes, it's Insulin.

That's right, it's elevated levels of insulin, and we talked a little bit about insulin's role in obesity in the last chapter. In fact, the obesity problem can be solved so easily, it is probably *the greatest* dietarily ignorant point I can highlight.

The problem with obesity is that it is the gateway to a host of diseases. Become obese and now you can hope for high blood pressure, diabetes, high cholesterol, high TGs, and a higher lifetime risk of cancer, just to name a few. In other words, while you do not have to be obese to develop these medical problems, if you are obese, you are at a greater risk for eventually developing either one or many of the diseases just mentioned.

So why is the obesity epidemic so easy to solve? You all know the answer by now. Obesity is due to elevated insulin levels. The higher one's insulin level, the more weight you gain; it's that simple.

Lower the insulin level, lower the obesity rate.

How do we lower insulin levels?

By lowering your carb intake.

I cannot make this any simpler.

Really, I can't.

"But hey, wait a minute," some of you may say, "I know people who eat all the carbs and sugar they want and they aren't overweight. Explain that to me."

Well, it's simple. Not everyone who overeats carbs squirts out a lot of insulin. And the genetics for obesity need to be present in order for one to gain weight while over consuming carbs. This means that your genetic blueprint must be such that your body is told, in the presence of insulin, to store carbs in the form of excess fat on the body. Not everyone's genetics tell their body to do this, which is why there are people out there who appear to get away with indulging in carbs, and they don't get fat.

We envy these people, we wish we were them. Well, guess what? Do not wish you were them because their genetics have other things in store for them. If your genetics are not telling your body to become overweight when insulin is around, then other signals, like make more cholesterol or TGs could be the result. I always tell my patients, if they point to the mildly overweight person and then to the obese person and ask me who's going to have the heart attack; my answer; I will point to the mildly overweight person. This is because the obese person's genetics are usually not such where a heart attack is right around the corner. But a heart attack is a few blocks away, unfortunately, for the obese individual.

The obese person's genetics are telling them to become obese. While it is true that obese people are at risk for heart disease, it is only after these people have become obese and have been obese for years that they start manifesting heart complaints in addition to other diseases.

The mildly overweight patient tends to have the heart attack a lot sooner because their genetics are telling their bodies to put plaque on their arterial walls, not to become obese. Instead of becoming visibly heavier, their genetics are telling them to become, shall I say, invisibly heavier. In a sense that arterial plaque buildup is only seen when it is looked for, either directly through a catheterization, or indirectly through a cardiac stress test. Just looking at someone who is mildly overweight will not tell you if they are at risk for a heart attack. So be careful judging a book by its cover.

But what if I'm not obese and I have clean arteries, then I'm in the clear, right?

Wrong?

Your genetics may be sending the signal when it sees insulin to create high blood pressure, or develop cancer. Let's not forget about allergies and asthma, irritable bowel disease, rheumatoid arthritis, acid reflux disease, pain, depression, and the list goes on. I will be talking about these diseases and their relationship to carb intake later in this book.

That's right, what disease you will see when your insulin levels are high depends upon your genetics. Unfortunately, doctors and scientists are way to ignorant to even offer an idea as to what disease you will see, until we see it. Even having defined the full genetic code, it means nothing because now we have to learn how to read it. And the story is different for each and every one of us. Even for identical twins.

Now I want to take the time to go over something we already discussed. Hopefully, I was able to help you understand why the calorie is a myth. You know what a myth is, Santa Claus, unicorns and fairies under the garden. Just to refresh, we spoke about how the calorie is a measurement that takes place in a closed system, where everything is known and how our bodies are open systems. One cannot relate an open to a closed system, for in open systems, too many things are going on for us to keep track of.

The reason obesity continues is largely in part to the belief that the calorie really means something. It does not. To reiterate, the term calorie is irrelevant as it is applied to human nutrition. If you want to know how much heat is given off when you burn, I mean literally burn your food; then you can use the calorie to define that. If you want to know what is really going to happen when you eat your food, we need to get rid of the term calorie. Period. Do not even allow yourself to use or say or think in terms of calories ever again.

Dietary ignorance plays a part when doctors believe the calorie is the Holy Grail of dieting and will solve all our problems. Just burn more calories than you eat and you will lose weight. How many obese people reading this book have done just that and not lost weight? Come on, hands up. I know there are millions of you. Probably the vast majority of overweight to obese people have tried this caloric restriction thing and it did not work.

You want to know why?

It's because if you continue to eat too may carbs, you continue to send all the signals to the body to not lose weight, but to gain weight. The more carbs we eat, the more insulin is secreted. The more insulin secreted, the more your body wants to maintain or gain weight. The whole burn more, eat less calorie mumbo jumbo has got to go. If it worked, well, there would be a lot less heavy people out there.

Well, I'll concede on one point. If you completely starve someone, as was my experience as a child, they'll lose weight. And if you're lucky, they won't die. Problem is when you starve someone they do not lose fat first. First to burn are your glycogen stores in your liver and muscle. Next, a little fat will be burned to replace those depleted glycogen stores. But the body soon figures out it isn't going to eat anytime soon and puts a stop to the burning of fat. This is called starvation mode. When this happens, your body starts to burn lean body tissue, like muscle, for fuel. This is not good.

Start burning muscle for fuel and now you become weaker. Oh, and your heart's a muscle, do you want to burn *that* for energy? Good answer. You don't! So burning muscle is not a good idea and starvation diets are not realistic ways to lose weight. So don't try them.

I must before I end this chapter talk about diet pills as weight loss aides. They are anything but.

Remember phen-fen, or was it fen-phen? Yes, this was the combining of two pills to help with weight loss. Oh yeah, this combo helped suppress appetite and people lost some weight; but many also developed an irreversible heart condition known as pulmonary hypertension.

As an aside, it was referred to as primary pulmonary hypertension in the literature, but that was incorrect. It should have been referred to as secondary pulmonary hypertension because it was second to something else, that is, the diet pills.

Problem with pulmonary hypertension is that it shortens your life expectancy, even after you stop the pills, which means you may lose some weight, but you will not be around long enough to enjoy it.

And then there was Meridia. To the doctors still reading this book, check out Meridia's molecular structure and compare it to fen-phen. Look similar? Hmmmm. Since I do not know of any reports of Meridia causing irreversible heart issues, I'll just say that using Meridia is still not a good idea because you are not overweight due to a deficiency of Meridia.

Ahhh, then there was Ma Huang and a host of other 'metabolic enhancers.' I love the marketing jargon, metabolic enhancers. Well who do the sellers of these bogus products think their kidding? Unfortunately, many of you. Billions of dollars are spent on these products each year in the hope that weight will be lost, or energy will be restored. Trust me, they do not work.

Oh yeah, by the way, Ma Huang is now off the market as it was killing people. Some people can get this stuff online and I wonder what they're actually getting. And besides, if someone has died as a result of using a particular over the counter product, why in the world would anyone want to even consider trying it to lose weight.

People try diet pills and will continue to try them in the hopes of quick weight loss. It's not really surprising that millions of these products are sold as millions of people either are, or think, they are overweight. Before physicians wave our fingers and ask why so many people want a quick fix, wasn't it doctors who started this whole quick fix thing in the first place. Of course the drug companies are guilty too, as they are more concerned with their profit margins.

The last medication for weight loss we really need to discuss is a medication that has been around for a while. This medication acts as a fat blocker. What do you think I'm going to say; that's right, you are not overweight because you're deficient in a fat blocker. Of course you're not.

Fat blocking meds should not be used for weight loss and can have dangerous side effects as well. Any physician who prescribes these medications has a profound misunderstanding of what causes us to become overweight in the first place.

You have enough information to explain to me why fat blocking meds should not be used, but allow me to take you through the thinking process as well. Remember, I make a conscious effort to be conscious everyday. Let's see how logical you find my reasoning.

Fat blocking meds block fat absorption. The fat being blocked is the fat found in the foods we eat. But what did we already learn about weight gain? We learned that we gain weight because of the presence of *insulin* in our blood. We also learned that eating fat would not make you fat, as long as your carb intake is low.

So the creator of this fat blocker medication, which by the way has renewed its advertising campaign, has produced a product which is absolutely worthless. Blocking fat will not have any appreciable effect on weight loss. Oh sure, the data which the drug company will show you will reveal remarkable weight loss trends. I'd like to see the data a year, even two years out. I have to admit that I have not even bothered to peruse the data, because the mechanism of action of these fat blockers immediately tells me the drug company has not a clue what causes one to gain weight.

What's worse, if it can get any worse, is that these fat blockers can inhibit the absorption of fat-soluble vitamins. The fat-soluble vitamins are vitamins A, D, E and K. If this happens, severe metabolic disturbances will occur. Not may, will. The fat blockers also can cause severe bloating, cramping and diarrhea; which is why a lot of people do not remain on these products.

But it gets better, or shall I say worse. In the brochure it actually states that if you're taking the fat blocker, you shouldn't eat over a certain amount of fat grams per day.

So now I'm really confused. The drug company markets a product, which is a fat blocker, but tells you not to eat fat. So what are we actually blocking here?

I'll tell you what we're blocking. We're blocking the absorption of important vitamins and causing belly pain, cramping and diarrhea, all because a drug company does not have a clue as to what is causing people to be over weight.

Once again, we become over weight because of the presence of insulin in our bloodstreams. Insulin levels become raised when we eat carbs. Lower your carb intake and you will lower your insulin level. Lower your insulin level and you will lose weight.

It really is that simple.

It has to be, because even I understand it.

CHAPTER TWENTY-DIABETES

There are at least two different types of diabetes. There is the Type I diabetic who requires insulin to survive, and then there is the Type II diabetic who actually has high insulin levels in their bloodstream. While the majority of this chapter will focus on Type II diabetics, I will also discuss Type I diabetes and how low carbs will help Type I diabetics as well.

Type II diabetes represents ninety to ninety-five percent of the diabetes in America. There are at least twenty million Type II diabetics in America, with this number varying depending on what study you read. The drug companies are working feverishly trying to find newer and better medications to control Type II diabetes.

Well, what if I were to tell you that we already have a cure for Type II diabetes?

Would you believe me?

What would you say if I told you I have treated thousands of Type II diabetics and have been able to keep the vast majority of Type II diabetics *off* medications?

Would you believe me?

What if I were to tell you the cure for Type II diabetes is not a pill, but in the foods we eat?

Again, would you believe me?

Of course the drug companies want you, and your physician, to believe the only way we'll get type II diabetes under control is through medications.

This is false.

By lowering one's carb intake, dramatic reductions in blood sugar occur, and many, if not all, of the type II diabetics who lower their carb intake rarely need medications. Through the lowering of one's carbs I have seen the average sugar, that is, the Hemoglobin A1c (or HgBA1c for short); go from a thirteen to a six in as little as four months. The greatest drop I've seen was from fifteen to under six in approximately four months. This same person started with a blood sugar over five hundred, and dropped his blood sugar to two hundred and fifty in two days and then to the one hundred fifty range in a few weeks. This is how quick a low carb diet will influence blood sugar numbers.

This is no joke.

Once the HgBA1c is under six the sugar is now considered in the normal range. Since most of the complications of the type II diabetic are due to an elevated blood sugar, then if the sugar is normal, the complications from an elevated blood sugar are eliminated. Complications also occur due to the elevated levels of insulin in the type II diabetic. This is why doctors must lower both the sugar *and* insulin levels, because elevated sugar and insulin levels cause tissue, and eventually, organ damage.

Type II diabetes used to be called maturity onset diabetes. This was because we did not see this type of diabetes until one hit their fifties or sixties. This has all changed. We are now seeing type II diabetes in persons under the age of twenty and even in children less than ten. The reason is due to the over consumption of carbohydrates.

We spoke about the possible pre-programming of the pancreas during embryological and fetal development in the pregnancy chapter. Just to refresh, it was my supposition that the developing baby's pancreas may become pre-programmed to over secrete insulin at a very early developmental age. If the baby's pancreas continues to see an elevated blood sugar in utero (in utero simply means when the baby is still in the uterus), the pancreas will always be secreting more insulin than it was biologically supposed to.

Unfortunately, most babies today are formula fed. Formula contains more sugar and less fat and cholesterol than breast milk. Formulas contain more sugar and less fat and cholesterol because the makers of formulas also think eating fat and cholesterol is bad. So our children are set up for the development of many medical problems not only in the womb, but after they are born as well. So the baby continues to see more sugar even after being born, because it is being fed a high sugar containing formula, and the baby's pancreas will continue to secrete more insulin than it should.

So whether the developing or newborn baby's pancreas is pre-programmed or not, the baby's pancreas will continue to secrete more insulin because it is continuously exposed to elevated levels of carbs. A pancreas can only make and secrete so much insulin, either at once or over the lifetime of the pancreas. If the pancreas cannot keep up its insulin secretion in response to a sugar load, the blood sugar level will then begin to rise. This is because the pancreas is at its maximum for insulin secretion and can secrete no more insulin. Once the blood sugar starts to rise because the pancreas cannot secrete any more insulin, type II diabetes begins.

Remember though, the child's pancreas from the get go, even while developing in the womb, was already making and secreting too much insulin. So now we have a child who is, say, nine years old and this nine year old's pancreas has been making and secreting elevated levels of insulin for nine years. This pancreas is tired. It cannot make any more insulin It has been making and secreting elevated levels of insulin for nine long years. The result, as stated above, is that blood sugars start to rise because the pancreas cannot produce any more insulin, and now you have diabetes in a nine year old.

There was something called the Hayflick constant that I learned about in undergraduate biology. This was a mathematical figure that represented how many times a cell can reproduce before it dies. When a cell dies, well, it's dead, and the cell cannot carry on any more of its functions.

I often wonder if this Hayflick constant can be applied to the cells of the pancreas which produce insulin. How long can these insulin-producing cells make and secrete large amounts of insulin? At what point do these cells just tire and die off, unable to produce insulin any further? The type II diabetic will eventually lose their ability to create insulin. Even though the type II diabetic started out with an elevated insulin level, eventually the insulin levels drop because the pancreas can no longer make any more insulin. It is at this point that the type II diabetic has now become a type I diabetic, and will require insulin shots to help control their blood sugar.

I bring this up because I am very concerned about the type II diabetes that is being seen in our children and adolescents. If type II diabetes is showing up this early, how long will these pancreases be able to make and secrete insulin?

Does this mean that we will start to see more insulin requiring diabetics, due to the insulin cells tiring and dying off at an even earlier age? Say, at age twenty-five or thirty? I'm not sure, but I am concerned that this will eventually happen. And nothing will get any better until the powers that be wake up and realize that low fat, low cholesterol diets are wrong. Dead wrong. And now our children are affected by this dietary ignorance.

Shouldn't that be enough?

How many more millions of people will die, or have to live with the complications of low fat, low cholesterol diets, before everyone finally knows the correct information about diets?

Why is it only a small, very small percentage of docs know that low carb diets are the correct way to eat and that following a low fat, low cholesterol diet is deadly?

I do not know, but I hope the powers-to-be realize they are wrong soon.

I remember growing up and hearing my doctor say that you could not get diabetes from eating too much sugar.

I'm here to tell you this isn't true. If we eat enough sugar we can gain weight. Once we start to gain weight our bodies become less sensitive to insulin. This is called insulin resistance. Insulin resistance means insulin cannot bring sugar into our cells as effectively. If less sugar is brought into our cells, more sugar will remain outside the cells. More sugar remaining outside the cells is exactly what diabetes is all about.

It is important to understand that both the elevated insulin and elevated blood sugar levels will cause the organ damage one sees all too frequently in diabetics. The classic organs which are damaged include the eyes (causing blindness), kidneys (which may require dialysis) and lower extremities (requiring possible amputation due to gangrene).

Remember the type II diabetic has elevated levels of insulin in the bloodstream and our pancreas's can only make and secrete so much insulin over our pancreas's lifetime. Once the pancreas reaches its limit of production of insulin it can make no more, and blood sugars will continue to rise because the insulin level can no longer keep pace with the rising sugars. It is at this point that the person starts to have symptoms of diabetes. The scary thing about type II diabetes is that alot of people with this type of diabetes have had it for years and do not even know about it. We can walk around for years, possibly five to seven years and usually longer, with sugars in the two hundred range, which is quite high, and not have any symptoms.

One of the best predictors of elevated blood sugars I've come to realize over the years is urinating at night (referred to as nocturia). Now I'm not talking about once or twice, but if someone is getting up four, five or six times at night to urinate, something's up and these people need to be investigated.

In a type II diabetic the insulin level in the bloodstream is high. This is to be distinguished from the type I diabetic whose insulin level is low. In the type I diabetic the pancreas has lost its ability to produce insulin. We are not sure why, but we think it may be the result of either the body attacking its own cells (called auto-immune destruction), or possibly a viral infection attacking and destroying the cells in the pancreas that make insulin. Since the pancreas of a type I diabetic can no longer make insulin, insulin must be provided or the type I diabetic will die.

Type 1 diabetics also benefit from lowering their carbs. The lower the carb intake, the less insulin the type I diabetic will need. It is important to remember that both sugar *and* insulin damage cells. I repeat this because too many type I diabetics think by just giving themselves a little more insulin, they can have that doughnut. Well, the problem is when the doughnut is consumed the blood sugar will elevate, this elevated blood sugar will cause tissue damage. Now when more insulin is taken to help lower the elevated sugar caused by eating that doughnut, this insulin will also cause damage to the cells. So it is not a very good idea to have an elevated sugar *or* insulin level.

OK, let's get back to the type II diabetic.

I stated in the beginning of my book that I'm not convinced our blood cholesterols are elevated because we're deficient in a cholesterol lowering medication, or that our blood pressures were elevated because we are deficient in blood pressure lowering medications. The same can be said of the type II diabetic. The type II diabetic does not have elevated blood sugars because they are deficient in blood sugar lowering medications. The type II diabetic has elevated blood sugars because they are eating too many carbs.

It's that simple.

It is extremely important to state that type II diabetes is a result of the inability of particular people to deal with carbs. A type II diabetic does not have any issues with the consumption of protein, fat, or cholesterol. For a type II diabetic it's all about the carbs and sugars. Remember, I use those two interchangeably. When I place my diabetic patients on a low carb diet the blood sugars immediately drop. This happens within a few days of starting low carbs, often within the first twenty-four hours. When we eat protein, fat or cholesterol containing foods, blood sugars do not elevate, unless we are eating carbs along with them.

Now let's talk about what happens in most doctors' offices throughout America when a person is diagnosed with type II diabetes. And remember, more and more children and adolescents are being given this diagnosis as well, and these children represent the future of America.

When a person is diagnosed with type II diabetes they are immediately told to avoid sugar, which is correct. But then they are told that eating fruit is ok, which is wrong, and are also told to get their carbs from only complex carbohydrates.

Now what exactly is a complex carbohydrate? A complex carbohydrate is allegedly a food, which is supposed to release its sugar molecules slowly, over many hours. The problem is that when a type II diabetic eats a so-called complex carb, it keeps the sugar elevated for, guess what, a couple of hours and sometimes for days. This is because a complex carbohydrate contains millions of sugar molecules just waiting to be set free. For a type II diabetic no carb is safe to eat, be it simple or complex. The mantra I have my diabetic patients repeat for me is that sugar is sugar is sugar. The message is that all sugars, from any source, can create problems for a diabetic.

The best bet is to just avoid carbs, especially if you're a type II diabetic. Sometimes I will place my type II diabetics on medications like metformin to help lower the sugar level. I'll usually use metformin in my obese patients with diabetes. This medication tells the cells to use insulin more effectively and also slows down the liver's production of sugar. By the way, the main reason blood sugars are elevated in the morning in type II diabetics is due to the liver's creation of sugar.

The neat thing about metformin is that by allowing the insulin to be used more effectively, insulin levels will drop in the bloodstream. When this happens it makes it easier for our bodies to lose weight. I discussed insulin's role as an anabolic hormone earlier in this book. To refresh, an anabolic hormone is something that makes things bigger, as in anabolic steroid. Insulin, as an anabolic hormone, allows us to get heavier. Type IIs, having a higher insulin level in the bloodstream, tend to almost always be overweight, and it is difficult for them to lose weight as well.

This is a catch 22 situation because in order to lose weight, one must lower the insulin level. But the type II diabetic has an elevated insulin level. So what can we do to help the type II diabetic lose weight? The answer is that we need to lower the insulin level in the type II diabetic. The best way to lower the insulin level, is, again, to lower the carb consumption, and the carbs need to be lowered dramatically. Also, by telling the liver to make less sugar, this will drop the amount of insulin secreted by the pancreas, and allows our bodies to continue to lose weight. Metformin does both, that is, it lowers insulin level and sugar production, which is why I find it useful. And eventually my patients are able to stop metformin, and stay off it, so long as they continue following a low carb regimen.

To recap, by lowering the carbs the pancreas squirts out less insulin. Less insulin traveling in the blood, the easier it becomes to lose weight. Once the weight comes off, the body starts to use the insulin more effectively and the blood sugars continue to normalize. Eventually, even if meds have been started to help lower the sugar (i.e. metformin), the meds can be stopped and the sugars will remain under control without medication. This can occur in a type II diabetic only, as the type I will always need to take insulin.

It cannot be overemphasized how important it is to lower the carb intake if you are a type II diabetic. One of the best books out there that anyone with diabetes or anyone who cares for diabetics should read is *Dr. Bernstein's Diabetes Solution,* by Richard K. Bernstein. I have found the guidelines in this book very useful and have been implementing Dr. Bernstein's dietary plan into my diabetic patient's lives for over seven years, with phenomenal success.

I have had many wonderful success stories with my diabetics who begin low carb diets. As described above, as soon as one starts to lower carbs the sugars immediately drop into the normal range. Most of my type II diabetics do not even need any diabetic meds as their sugars are very well controlled without medications. I still get excited when sugars normalize without medications and I have seen this time and again for over nine years. The best thing about normalizing the blood sugar is that once the sugars are normalized, one will not have to worry about medical issues such as dialysis, gangrene (with the associated amputations) or blindness. The medical problems associated with diabetes result from the sugar *and* insulin being elevated. Once the sugar and insulin levels become normal, the type II diabetic cannot suffer from these debilitating and deadly diabetic complications. I know the insulin levels normalize as I check insulin levels too, and can see the insulin levels drop along with the blood sugars.

I must mention as a safety note that if you are taking meds like Glucotrol, Glipizide, or Amaryl (the so-called sulfonylureas), lowering your carb intake without first consulting a doctor who knows how to implement low carbs, could be very dangerous. Doing so could result in death. It is because these medications lower the blood sugar no matter what. So once the carbs are lowered these medications will continue to lower the blood sugar number, no matter how low the blood sugar number is at the time, and can lower it to a life threatening value. This is why it is imperative to lower your carb intake only under the guidance of a clinician with low carb experience.

For my patients who come in on these medications, as I rarely, if ever, prescribe them; I will usually instruct them that if their blood sugars drop under a hundred on three consecutive occasions, they are to stop those medications. This prevents the blood sugars from dropping dangerously low. I also tell my patients to set their alarm clock to two or three am in the morning and check their sugar values to make sure they are not falling too low.

Another reason I do not like using meds like Glucotrol or glipizide is because they work by stimulating the pancreas to secrete insulin. You know by now that insulin is not a very safe thing to have floating around in our bloodstream in high amounts. In fact, there is a direct warning on the packaging label that states sulfonylureas can increase one's risk of heart disease. This should not come as a shock to anyone still reading as you now know that insulin plays a large part in the production of cholesterol, makes us fatter, causes cellular damage, and the list goes on.

A type I diabetic can also benefit from a low carb diet. However, they also need to be very careful and a constant monitoring of the blood sugar is mandatory, just like the type II. I will usually tell my type I's to cut their insulin in half as soon as they start low carbs, because the blood sugars start to drop immediately. I have seen dramatic effects even on brittle diabetics, with more stable blood sugar readings, reflected on a daily basis as well as within the HgBA1c readings. The most important thing for a type I diabetic to remember is that if the sugar is too low, the *insulin* dose needs to be lowered. If the sugar is dangerously low, say, under fifty, one can use glucose tablets to raise the sugar up in a controlled manner. I tell my patients to avoid drinking orange juice, or having a bunch of cookies, because then the sugar goes way too high. Again, the most important part of implementing a low carb diet is working with a clinician with experience in low carb diets.

I want to take time to discuss another very important and often misunderstood lab test that all diabetics should have. One of the routine labs doctors check is the microalbumin level in the urine. Albumin is a type of protein molecule. Since microalbumin is a protein, checking the microalbumin level will let physicians know if there is protein in the urine. If there is protein in the urine, known as microalbuminuria, it is an early warning sign that kidney damage may be occurring and allows doctors to start appropriate medications to protect the kidneys.

Now here's the problem with microalbuminuria. Yes, it is a measurement of how much protein is in the urine. Normally there should be very little protein in the urine. If the kidneys have suffered damage due to diabetes, there will be more protein found and the microalbumin level will be elevated. A common error that physicians make is in thinking that if the microalbumin level is high, this is due to the patient eating too much protein.

This is wrong.

The microalbumin level is high in the urine not because the patient is eating too much protein, but because the elevated sugar has damaged the filtration mechanism of the kidney. It is very important to understand that in order to halt and reverse this kidney damage, one must lower their *carbohydrate* intake, not their protein intake. Lowering protein in the diet will not reverse any damage which may have occurred or is occurring within the kidney, and will actually make it worse. This is because the damage was caused by the *elevated blood sugar* not by the protein in the diet. If one lowers their protein consumption, what do you think will take the place of the protein in the diet? That's right, carbohydrates; and it was the consumption of carbohydrates, coupled with the body's inability to handle those carbs, which led to the kidney damage in the first place. Microalbuminuria is due to carbohydrate over consumption, not protein. This point cannot be over emphasized.

If physicians just stopped and thought it through they would realize the kidney damage is caused by the sugar molecules binding to kidney cells, biochemically referred to as glycosylation. This messes up the function of the kidney cell, which is why more protein gets in the urine. Eating more protein will not cause more damage, nor will it increase the microalbumin level in the urine, because it was not the protein that caused any damage. I know this because I have been feeding my patients more protein with elevated microalbumins over nine years and I do not see a rise in the urinary microalbumins; so long as the carb intake is reduced as well.

This is another example of the dietary ignorance of physicians. I still get consultative reports from nephrologists stating that due to the elevated microalbumin levels in the urine, the patient was instructed to lower their protein intake. This is another example of a priori reasoning because the physician is equating the higher urinary protein levels, with dietary protein consumption. So the doctor incorrectly reasons that more protein is in the urine because one is eating more protein, which is not true. Again, more protein is in the urine because the kidney's filtration mechanism has been damaged due to elevated sugar levels in the blood stream. This is similar to the continued incorrect thinking that cholesterol and fats are elevated in the bloodstream because we're eating too much of those things in our diet.

And we now know that is wrong as well.

True, we like to think of things in simple terms and it would be easier clinically if the elevated protein levels in the urine were due to dietary intake of protein, but this is not true. In fact, as stated above, lowering one's protein intake almost certainly means greater intake of carbs, and it is the presence of the carbs that caused the damage in the first place. So, if we instruct a patient with microalbuminuria to lower their protein intake, *we will make things worse.* We are actually going to cause more kidney damage, not less.

What happens when I tell my diabetics with microalbuminuria to eat more protein and lower their carb intake, which is directly opposite to what the vast majority of specialists would recommend? Well, after recommending to my patients to eat less carbs and more protein, I have seen microalbumins in the one-hundred range go back to normal in approximately four months, once a low carb diet is started. These patients were eating more protein, not less, and their microalbumins still went back to normal. This is strong evidence that the microalbumins were elevated due to the *elevated sugar* causing the kidney damage, *not* the protein in the diet. This point is so important because if the doctor believes that eating more protein will increase the kidney damage, they will tell you to eat less protein. Well, if you're eating less protein, like I said above, guess what you're eating more of? That's right---carbs! And, once again, it was the carbs that caused the damage in the first place. So by following the advice of your well intentioned doctor, who by the way may be your endocrinologist, internist, family doc or nephrologist, or, even sadly enough, your pediatrician; you will actually cause more kidney damage, resulting in the possible need for dialysis in the future. How's that for dietary ignorance?

OK, let's leave diabetes and talk about more diseases which lowering one's carb intake will help. The next two chapters will discuss how lowering your carbs helps decrease your risk of coronary artery disease and how it helps to control your blood pressure.

CHAPTER TWENTY-ONE-CORONARY ARTERY DISEASE (CAD)

CAD is the number one killer of both men and women in the United States. We already learned how our bodies make cholesterol. We spoke about how our bodies make cholesterol out of the very foods that contain **no** cholesterol. We discussed that if we eat cholesterol-containing foods, our bodies **make even less** cholesterol and actually stop making the very thing our bodies need (HMG CoA reductase) to manufacture cholesterol.

CAD continues to be the number one killer because of the widespread belief that low fat, low cholesterol diets are safe and effective.

They are not.

If they were, we should be seeing lower rates of CAD, as many Americans pride themselves on the fact they are following a low fat, low cholesterol diet. But CAD rates continue to increase, as has the use of all types of cardiac medications.

My critics will immediately state that the reason we are using more cardiac meds is because our population is living longer. While some of this may be true, could it also be that we are being exposed even longer to the wrong way of eating and stay behind the eight ball as long as we continue to follow a low fat, low cholesterol diet?

Low fat, low cholesterol diets are killing and continue to kill, and handicap, millions of Americans, and people worldwide each year. The longer low fat, low cholesterol diets are used in the hopes to lower heart disease, the longer we will continue to see more heart disease. Low fat, low cholesterol diets are the single biggest killer of Americans, and everyone else who follows them. Period.

So if you want to die from heart disease, or a whole host of other medical diseases, follow a low fat, low cholesterol dietary regimen. There are plenty of guides out there. If you want to stay on this planet for as long as possible, immediately start to lower your carbs and increase your fat, cholesterol and protein content, but remember to only do this once you've found an experienced doctor who has used and understands low carb dieting. To repeat, if your doctor even makes a hint that low carb diets are bad, go out and find yourself a doctor who understands why low carb diets are safe and effective, and do it fast.

Getting back to heart disease, we probably all know some-one who has had a stent placed or has had a bypass graft performed. Doctors are also aware there is a risk of these stents and the bypasses becoming clogged again with cholesterol plaque, with the need for more stents or re-peat bypass operations to undue this reclogging. Now it should not come as a shock to anyone reading this book that the reason we see this re-occlusion (reclogging), is because of the ignorant dietary advice given to our heart patients when they are discharged from the hospital.

What do you think these patients are told dietarily when they are discharged from the hospital after having a stent or bypass graft performed? That's right, they are told to follow a low fat, low cholesterol diet. Now what do you think caused the initial clogging in the first place? That's right, a low fat, low cholesterol diet. So when our cardiac patients are discharged from the hospital after having a stent placed or a heart bypass graft performed, they are told to follow the same exact diet that got them to clog up their arteries in the first place.

Can I hear a great big OOOPPPS !!!!

Until doctors wake up and realize that they are giving the wrong dietary advice, we will continue to have to place stents and perform bypasses. Unless, of course, we succeed in wiping out the entire population of our planet with the ridiculous dietary advice doctors continue to give. Does this not constitute genocide?

To repeat an important point, when our cardiac patients are discharged and told to follow a low fat, low cholesterol diet, the dieticians do not think whole grains and fruits are dangerous. They feel these are natural foods and safe to eat. The trained nutritionists, dieticians, and doctors do not understand that sugar is sugar is sugar. They do not understand that our cells cannot distinguish where the sugar came from. They do not understand that at the cellular level when a cell sees sugar it will do what it does, no matter where the sugar molecule came from. If they did, and if everyone understood, especially physicians, that our bodies make cholesterol and fat out of the very things that do not contain cholesterol and fat, that is, carbs; no one would give the ridiculously ignorant dietary advice to follow a low fat, low cholesterol diet. But it continues to happen and will continue to happen until the people who provide us with our dietary information understand the dangers of low fat, low cholesterol diets.

Now let's look a little bit at what exactly CAD is, and how low carb diets help lower your risk, and quite substantially I might add. As the name suggests, CAD, or coronary artery disease, is a disease of the arteries that supply the heart itself with blood. Since the heart is a muscle it needs a blood supply to nourish it, and this blood supply is derived from the coronary arteries. If the coronary arteries become clogged with plaque, less blood is able to flow through these arteries, and less blood gets to the heart itself.

When blood flow to the heart is decreased, this is referred to as ischemia. If blood flow stops entirely, this is referred to as a heart attack (or myocardial infarction). The more plaque accumulating within the coronary arteries, the less blood flow to the heart, and this is what is meant by coronary artery disease.

Now it may come as a shock, even to my physician readers, that the cholesterol in the foods we eat has never, and I mean never, been shown to be the *same* cholesterol which clogs up our coronary arteries, or any other artery for that matter. This is extremely interesting and very important, because low fat, low cholesterol diets are based on this premise. But where did this premise come from? It all goes back to chapter one, a priori reasoning.

A priori reasoning says if your cholesterol is high, don't eat cholesterol; or if you're overweight, well, stop eating fat dummy. In the preceding chapters we have learned this reasoning does not work in regards to cholesterol and fat consumption. We have learned that our cholesterols are not elevated because we are eating cholesterol; in fact we now know that the more cholesterol one consumes in their diet, the more favorable your cholesterol profile will be. We also learned that we do not get fat from eating fat, as long as we're not over eating carbs in the process, and we now know it's very easy to over eat carbs. Doctors are still holding on tenaciously to the incorrect premise that our cholesterols are high because we are eating too much cholesterol, or we are fat because of too much fat consumption, and we've applied this incorrect premise to CAD as well.

Let's look at a priori reasoning as applied to CAD. It goes something like this; if our coronary arteries are clogged with cholesterol plaque, it must be that we ate and are eating too much cholesterol. A priori reasoning continues to lead us to the wrong conclusions. Unfortunately, in the case of CAD, it leads us to a deadly wrong conclusion, with emphasis on the dead.

While there have been no studies tracking the cholesterol in the foods we eat to see where it goes, we do know that all the carbon atoms that make up cholesterol come from acetyl CoA, which is derived from carbs. We all know where I am going with this one. We have no studies tracing where the cholesterol in the foods we eat goes to in our bodies; but we do have studies showing the entire cholesterol molecule can be derived from carbs; hmmmmm... interesting.

Now some of my readers who have dabbled a bit in biochemistry may immediately shoot back and say, "Hey, wait a minute, cholesterol in the foods we eat can also be broken down to acetyl Co A, and this can be used to make more cholesterol." I will respond by saying, good point, but they are forgetting about the negative biofeedback loop.

Remember that when we eat cholesterol we send signals throughout our bodies to stop making the things we need to make cholesterol. So, when we eat cholesterol we actually turn off the machinery to make cholesterol. So we will break down cholesterol in the foods we eat to acetyl Co A; but if the stuff isn't there to reassemble these acetyl things back into cholesterol, we cannot make cholesterol.

Again to my critics I say, please make your argument as to why low fat, low cholesterol diets are safe and that low carbs, more fat, more cholesterol and more protein diets are dangerous, and I can refute your argument, usually in under a minute, with factual biochemical and clinical data.

Another thing concerning CAD I need to address is the incorrect information some of my patients have been given in regards to low carb dieting. It goes something like this; a patient of mine comes in, I perform lab work and find out their HDL is low and TGs are high. I immediately place them on a low carb diet, and yes that means they are also eating more cholesterol, more fat and more protein. Then about a month, or two months later, this same patient has a heart attack. The cardiologist asks how they were eating and they tell the cardiologist they were eating low carbs, more cholesterol, more fat and more protein. The cardiologists says, "Ah hah, there you go, another example of why eating low carbs and more cholesterol is dangerous. See, eating that way caused you to have a heart attack." Or did it? Let's work through this ridiculously ignorant reasoning which happens every day in thousands of cardiologist, internist and family doctor's offices throughout America.

Ask any doctor how long it takes to build up plaques within your arteries and they will respond that the process takes many years. We are talking around twenty to thirty years, not a few months. What these cardiologists (and I really should not pick on the heart docs, because just about all docs are guilty of this line of reasoning) are forgetting is that it takes decades, not months, to build up enough plaque to cause a heart attack. To blame what someone has been doing for a few months and ignoring how he or she were eating for thirty years is irresponsible. In fact, it's downright ignorant. It was not the few months of eating low carbs that caused the heart attack; it was how the person was eating for the last thirty years that allowed the heart attack to occur.

When a few of my patients had the unfortunate experience of suffering a heart attack after being on low carbs for a few months, and were told the low carb diet did it, I picked up the phone with the patient present and called their cardiologist to ask the cardiologist some questions. It went something like this, and yes, I had the cardiologist on speakerphone with the patient present.

"Hi, doctor so and so, this is Dr Carlson calling, I just had a quick question to ask you."

"Uh, huh, go ahead."

"I was just wondering how long it takes, for say, cholesterol plaque to clog a coronary artery?"

The cardiologist responds, "Gosh, Jim, it takes at least twenty to thirty years for enough plaque to develop on a coronary artery to cause a heart attack."

(Now remember, the cardiologist is on speakerphone.)

So I say, "OK, so you're saying it takes about twenty to thirty years for enough plaque to develop on a coronary artery to cause a heart attack."

"That's right."

(Now the coup de grace.)

"Then why would you suggest to my patient that the way they were eating over the last few months, not the way they were eating over the last twenty to thirty years, caused their heart attack?"

The cardiologists have no response and a dial tone usually follows.

To sum up, CAD is the number one killer of people worldwide and CAD rates increase if one follows a low fat, low cholesterol diet. By following a low carb, more fat, more cholesterol, more protein diet, CAD rates will drop significantly. Also, by telling people who are discharged from the hospital after having a stent or heart bypass graft to follow low carbs, we will see less in the way of readmissions due to re-clogging of these stents and bypass grafts. Until all doctors and dietary advisors understand the dangers inherent in low fat, low cholesterol diets, CAD rates will continue to climb and we will never see a significant decrease in CAD.

Again, my critics will say we have seen a decrease in CAD and will prove this with statistical data. But this decrease

in CAD is not significant and it has all to do with the use
of medications.

How about this one? How about we significantly lower CAD
without using meds and do it naturally? It can be done, and
it can be accomplished through low carb dieting.

CHAPTER TWENTY-TWO-HYPERTENSION

Hypertension is just the fancy way doctors refer to high blood pressure. Most cases of high blood pressure are without any symptoms. This is why high blood pressure is referred to as the 'silent' killer. The silent refers to the absence of any symptoms which would warn you that you have high blood pressure, such as a headache or blurry vision. The killer part comes in when the high blood pressure remains undiagnosed over many years and one has a stroke, heart attack, or requires the need for dialysis. (About 25% of patients undergoing dialysis are there because of kidney damage caused by hypertension.)

Most people think that headaches, blurry vision, or nose bleeds suggests they have high blood pressure, but this is not true. When I take a blood pressure reading in my office and find it elevated, most patients do not want to believe it. They'll ask if I checked it right. Since I've checked tens of thousands of blood pressures over the last sixteen years, the answer is yes, I checked the blood pressure correctly. Or they'll come up with some excuse as to why their blood pressure is high; for example, hard day at work, kids are aggravating me, etc.

One of the scariest things about elevated blood pressure, as if stroke, heart attack or dialysis aren't scary enough, is that untreated blood pressure can cause a very similar dementia as is seen in Alzheimer's disease.

Alzheimer's disease is a severe, debilitating disease of the brain, which affects, initially, a patient's short-term memory capability. As the disease progresses, memories become worse and patients eventually return to a childlike state, where they are dependant upon others for help with basic activities of daily living.

If blood pressure goes untreated for many years, a multi-infarct dementia may occur, and clinically presents very similar to Alzheimer's disease. In fact, a clinician usually cannot tell which patient has memory issues because of Alzheimer's disease, and which patient has memory loss due to multi-infarct dementia. I will usually use the multi-infarct dementia example to, hopefully, get my patients to make sure their blood pressures are in the normal range.

So how do carbs affect one's blood pressure? I spoke a little bit about this in the pregnancy chapter, but let me reiterate some points further.

When we eat carbs, the carbs are broken down into sugar and sugar causes the pancreas to release insulin into the bloodstream. This scenario has been repeated quite often throughout this book. We have learned that insulin is necessary for our survival, and we have also learned that too much insulin causes bad things to happen to us as well.

Another bad thing insulin does is stimulate the growth of smooth muscle found within arteries, and the smaller arteries known as arterioles. When this smooth muscle grows it narrows the diameter of the artery. As the artery becomes narrower, the pressure will increase. This can be demonstrated quite easily by placing your thumb over the end of a garden hose. The more you prevent the water from coming out, by placing more thumb over the opening, the further you can squirt the water. This is because you are increasing the pressure, by narrowing the opening, which is exactly what happens to increase the blood pressure in our arteries.

The same thing happens when the smooth muscle narrows the diameter of the arteries and arterioles. This narrowing will increase the pressure in the artery and when this happens, high blood pressure will result. Having an elevated blood pressure will cause wear and tear on all the arteries and will place one at risk for strokes, heart attacks, kidney problems, vision issues and multi-infarct dementia, as described above. It should not come as a shock that insulin causes the growth of smooth muscle, because we have already mentioned insulin's role as an anabolic hormone. Remember that the term anabolic means growth.

I also have more questions than I can answer about this smooth muscle growth due to insulin's presence. Does this growth happen in utero, when our babies are in the womb, if too much insulin is secreted? If it does, will this set-up our children for blood pressure problems at a younger age?

I am seeing more children and adolescents with elevated blood pressures. Is this the reason?

Another interesting thing insulin does is that it tells the kidney to hold on to more salt and not let it get into our urine. In clinical talk, it increases the absorption of salt at the level of the kidney and less salt is excreted, or passed out of the body. The result is an elevated salt level in the bloodstream. The more salt that is retained, the more fluid is retained because salt attracts water; or water loves salt, however you want to look at it. We all know this because when we eat something salty, we get thirsty and want to chug some water. So the end result of more salt in the body is more water in body. More water in the body means more fluid in our arteries. More fluid in our arteries, the higher the blood pressure. Don't forget that this also means there is more fluid in a narrowed artery, so this drives up blood pressures even further.

To recap, insulin will not only narrow our arteries, causing an elevated blood pressure, but will cause us to retain more salt leading to a further elevation in blood pressure. How do we control this? By controlling the amount of insulin released by our pancreas. How do we control the amount of insulin released by our pancreas? Lower the carb intake. I think you get it by now.

It is because of insulin that one week we'll hear salt is bad and then another week we'll hear salt may not be as bad. If one is following a low carb diet, even if one consumes too much salt, the body will get rid of the salt in the urine. This is because there is not a lot of insulin around telling our kidneys to retain the salt. In the study suggesting salt is bad, the participants were following a low fat, low choles-terol diet and eating too many carbs. The carbs will cause an increase in insulin secretion and now the kidney will hold on to the salt. This will elevate the blood pressure.

I still tell my patients to watch their salt intake, but they don't get into too much trouble if they have a little more salt than they should, since they are eating low carbs, and are able to get rid of the salt in their urine.

CHAPTER TWENTY-THREE
GASTROESOPHAGEAL REFLUX DISEASE (GERD) & IRRITABLE BOWEL DISEASE (IBD)

This will be a very interesting chapter for the millions of people suffering from gastro esophageal reflux and irritable bowel diseases. To save my calloused fingers a little bit, I will use the abbreviations, GERD and IBD, for these two diseases in this chapter.

GERD is a condition that affects millions of us. There is a billion dollar drug industry devoted to medications to treat the symptoms of GERD. There are even over the counter meds that people can use as well. I will refrain from mentioning any of these meds because I am not here to adver tise for the drug companies. In fact, with the information contained in this chapter, most of you suffering from GERD or IBD may be able to stop your medications. If that doesn't excite you, think of the drug co-pays you'll save. If you are someone who is lucky enough to have good insurance (is 'good insurance' considered an oxymoron), and has low co-pays for any medications, I offer you this; even if your symptoms disappear while taking your anti-reflux medication, the reflux may still be there causing damage to the lining of your esophagus. You will not have any symptoms because the medication is not allowing you to feel anything. As long as the reflux continues, and you don't know this because you're not feeling it, the damage continues, and cancer may be the end result. Yes, I did use the 'c' word. This is why this chapter is so important for you GERD sufferers.

Also, persons with reflux are at risk for strictures developing where the esophagus meets the stomach.

As an aside, the esophagus is what I like to call the food tube. When we eat or drink, what allows food and liquid to get into the stomach is the esophagus, which connects the mouth to the stomach.

These strictures, if severe enough, can prevent food and liquids from getting into the stomach. If food is prevented from getting into the stomach, special tubes have to be inserted to open up this narrowing. No, it isn't a pleasant procedure.

It is important to mention that I am referring to GERD and IBD only; I am not talking about those of you who had or have had bleeding ulcers, be it stomach or small intestinal (duodenal). You need to stay on your meds, as they will help heal your ulcer. In addition, those of you who have the Helicobacter pylori infection in the stomach, also need to stay on your meds to help with healing. This chapter is only dealing with GERD and IBD sufferers.

Now what do you think I'm going to tell you GERD sufferers to do? You gals and guys are getting good; that's right, lower your carb intake. There is a word out there known as serendipity. Serendipity is the act of discovering something by accident. The alleviation of the symptoms of GERD, due to following a low carb diet, was definitely a serendipitous moment of mine.

In my introduction I mentioned that when I was following the low fat, low cholesterol diet, I had to start cholesterol and blood pressure lowering medications. What I left out was that I also took antacids as I suffered from severe heartburn. My heartburn was so bad I would be doubled over with pain and had to stop whatever I was doing until the antacid kicked in. I took so much in the way of antacids I was peeing chalk. OK, I wasn't really urinating chalk, but you get my point.

Ahhh, then I started lowering my carbs and guess what happened. That's right, the heartburn went away, almost immediately. I didn't really put two and two together right away, remember, I am a physician. It wasn't until I ate more carbs then I should have and the heartburn came right back, that I then made the connection.

Armed with this new knowledge, I began to tell my patients with GERD to lower their carbs. Guess what happened? For those patients who listened to my advice, their heartburn immediately went away. I'm talking within a week, most of my patients who significantly lowered their carbs were off their antacid medications, and feeling a lot better. Again, I only instructed my patients with definitive

GERD, who had no known ulcers that it was alright to stop their antacids. My patients who had bleeding ulcers were also told to start lowering their carbs, but were told to NOT stop taking their meds as antacids are curative for those with bleeding ulcers, and should not be stopped unless under the guidance of their belly doctor (that is, their gastroenterologist, but I like belly doctor because it's easier to say).

Now, nine years after using low carb diets in my practice, I routinely counsel my patients with GERD to lower their carbs. Again, when my patients listen, the large majority are able to stop their antacid meds. This includes prescription antacid medications. If someone is able to stay off the antacid meds and not experience any symptoms of heartburn, they can be rest assured they are not having any major reflux. No major reflux, no continuous damage to the esophagus's lining. No continuing damage to the esophagus's lining means there is a much lower chance of getting esophageal cancer, or the more common strictures, which are both created by the continuous reflux.

By the way, people get these strictures even on antacid meds. Why? As mentioned above, even if the person does not have any symptoms, reflux can still be occurring and you will not know this because the medication is masking the symptoms. Since one may still have reflux, even on prescription antacid medications, continuous irritation to the lower part of the esophagus occurs, and this is exactly what causes the strictures.

It is extremely interesting that one of the reasons the medical profession did not want prescription antacids to go over the counter, is because we know that symptom relief does not mean the reflux has stopped. The doctors knew that if one is on antacids the disease could still be creating problems, such as strictures, or setting one up for cancer, even if no symptoms were present. Funny thing is, some doctors still prescribe antacids and believe symptom relief means the disease has gone away. This is not true and unfortunately it represents another area of ignorance for doctors.

The fact of the matter is that if a patient with GERD is told to lower their carb intake, their GERD will go away.

Individuals who start low carb diets will not only experience symptom relief, but the disease will go away. The drug companies who make antacid products cannot claim this. The meds only diminish the symptoms, and I used the word diminish on purpose because most people still have some symptoms of reflux even while on antacids.

I know, I know, some of you docs and even drug companies will say I cannot provide clinical proof of what I am saying. My evidence is clinical experience, as my patients on low carb diets do not experience any symptoms of GERD. None at all. Which will surprise a lot of docs, and most people reading this, because isn't the consumption of fat and cholesterol suppose to cause really bad heartburn?

This is a very important point to be made because it is not the fat or cholesterol containing food that is causing the heartburn; it is the food which contains the carbs. So, it is not the sausage or meatballs which upsets the belly, it is the pasta. It is not the steak; it is the corn and mash potatoes. It is not the eggs; it is the pancake or hash browns. We have become so accustomed to blaming the wrong food items for heartburn; it has now become common nature to blame the wrong food. I hear docs blaming the wrong food all the time.

You can prove it to yourself by eliminating the carbs and see what happens to the heartburn. I'll let you be the judge. Not to be annoying, but just to make sure you are all safe, remember, if you are on meds for a bleeding ulcer, do not stop them to test out what I'm saying, you can start to bleed again, and this can kill you. You have been warned.

Let me now talk a little bit about irritable bowel disease or syndrome. Commonly referred to as IBD, or IBS, this is another condition which affects millions of people. This was also another serendipitous finding, because when I started my IBD patients on low carbs for other reasons, they began experiencing less symptoms of IBD. Since I was primed from my initial ignorance of low carb's effect on GERD, I was more open to any possible connection between the lowering of carbs and symptom relief for any disease process.

IBD is notoriously difficult to treat. It is a terrible condition which limits the ability of persons afflicted to carry on simple activities of daily living. When people with IBD eat, they almost immediately have to run to the bathroom to have a bowel movement. As one might imagine, if this happens after every time one eats, it can really affect your day.

Unfortunately, it's not just the running to the bathroom that gets in the way, there's also an ever-present pain all over the belly and a lot of gas and cramping. So when an IBD sufferer isn't in the bathroom, they are still experiencing other effects of the disease. This can and does totally interfere with the life of the person with IBD.

The common treatment for an IBD patient is to start medications known as selective serotonin re-uptake inhibitors. This is only after the person goes through a complete work-up, often in conjunction with a gastroenterologist, and other diseases have been ruled out. These medications are effective as the belly and intestines are known to have many serotonin receptors. I, too, use these medications, and continue to use these meds, to help my IBD patients lead a more normal life.

When I began low carb diets for my patients who had IBD for other reasons, that is, to help lower TGs or blood sugars, a remarkable thing happened. Most, if not all, of the symptoms resolved. This included the rushing to the bathroom, the belly pain and the associated gas and bloating. The symptoms went away so much, that if a particular patient happened to be on a med for their IBD, some were able to stop their meds. I now routinely recommend to my patients with IBD to try a low carb diet, before any medications. For those patients who try the low carbs, they are very happy with the outcome.

Unfortunately, having an IBD patient start a low carb diet is difficult, as the IBD sufferer fears and thinks any food they eat will cause them to have symptoms. I counsel my patients that lowering the carbs will have other health benefits, so just give it a try and see what you think. Most of my IBD patients who honestly try low carbs are very happy with the results, and rarely go back to eating more carbs.

CHAPTER TWENTY-FOUR-MISCELLANEOUS DISEASES

COLITIS

Colitis refers to a severe inflammation of both the small and large intestines. Colitis is not GERD or IBD. Colitis causes severe, incapacitating abdominal pain, bloody diarrhea, weight loss, anemia, and the list goes on. This serious affliction can occur in any age group, even in children as young as two. It is diagnosed by performing a colonoscopy, which will demonstrate an 'ulcerative pattern' seen within the large intestine. Depending upon the distribution of these ulcers, the patient will be diagnosed with either Crohn's or Ulcerative colitis. These are diseases where lowering carbs will help with some of the symptoms, but patients usually need to continue on the anti-inflammatory meds, as prescribed by their gastroenterologist.

I began to institute low carbs in patients with colitis after I made the connection between carbs and inflammation. My reasoning was that since colitis is a disease of inflammation and since it is known biochemically that eating carbs can increase inflammation; wouldn't it make sense that the inflammation we see in colitis could be lessened by lowering the carb intake?

In Part 1 of this book I spoke of a thing known as arachidonate. Arachidonate was released in the second messenger system by insulin's action on our cells. Since carbs cause insulin secretion to occur in the first place, which then causes more arachidonate to be created, could lowering one's carb intake influence the amount of arachidonate produced? And since arachidonate produces the very things that allow us to feel pain, that is, prostaglandins, could lowering the amount of arachidonate, lower the creation of the very things we need to feel pain?

Since by this time I had gained a lot of experience with low carb diets, and felt comfortable with the safety of starting people on low carbs, I began to suggest to those patients with colitis to lower their carb intake. When my patients with colitis lowered their carb intake, most experienced less abdominal pain. While most patients had to continue with their anti-inflammatory meds, the vast majority had a lessening of their pain and they were able to function better throughout the day.

Critics may say colitis is a medical disease and lowering the carbs will have no influence, but I disagree. The fact that most patients experienced a lessening of their symptoms where they were able to function better throughout the day, after lowering their carb intake, speaks highly in favor for the introduction of a low carb diet into patient's lives with colitis. I continue to make this suggestion in my daily practice, and again, most patients are grateful due to the symptom relief they experience.

ECZEMA PSORIASIS ALLERGIES ASTHMA

It may seem a little weird that skin conditions, asthma or allergies would respond to a low carb diet. This was another serendipitous finding after I began incorporating low carbs into my patient's lives. The low carb diet was started because of some other medical reason, usually high TGs or low HDL; the most common things I see in my office.

Interestingly enough, when patients with eczema or psoriasis began a low carb regimen, their skin conditions got better, and some patients had complete resolution of symptoms. By this point in my low carb career, I knew all about how both these skin conditions were a result of inflammatory and/or allergic processes within the skin. Psoriasis is more inflammatory, whereas eczema is more allergic. Knowing about arachidonate and about how this substance breaks down to create both inflammatory and allergy provoking byproducts, I was not all that surprised when these two skin conditions were helped by the introduction of a low carb diet.

I also wondered if the introduction of more fat was helpful because along with the lowering of carbs, fat intake also increases. I'm not sure which helped more? Was it mainly the lowering of the carbs; or was it a combination of lowered carbs, along with the consumption of more fat, cholesterol and protein? In any event, the fact remains that these two skin conditions are definitely helped with low carb, more fat, more cholesterol and more protein diets. (Just to remind everyone, notice how I am not saying *no* carb, *high* fat, *high* cholesterol, *high* protein, because that is *not* the diet I am talking about here.)

For you critics out there we spoke about the inflammatory promoting aspect of arachidonate. We also spoke about how arachidonate can be broken down to create things referred to as leukotrienes, which are known chemical mediators for allergies. In fact, there exist prescription drugs that are leukotriene inhibitors, which we doctors use in severe allergic conditions and asthma. It makes perfect sense if we decrease the amount of leukotrienes our bodies normally produce, we can lessen, and possible eliminate, allergic symptoms.

Since I have placed thousands of patients on low carb diets over the last nine years, I have definitely had a number of patient's state their allergic symptoms have diminished, and some were even able to stop their allergy meds. This holds true, too, for those patients who suffered from psoriasis and eczema.

In asthma, patients did claim a reduction in symptoms, but I still cautioned my patients to carry their rescue inhalers with them, just in case. Those of my patients on inhaled steroids coupled with other meds were cautiously weaned, to see if a rescue puff or two was needed. Those who needed to use their rescue inhaler on a daily basis, despite being on low carbs, were told to continue with their maintenance inhalers. Again, it must be stressed, that most of my asthmatic patients on low carb diets did notice a reduction in symptoms. No, lowering the carbs did not solve all the asthmatic's problems, but it sure did help. Also, the longer one stays on a low carb regimen, asthmatic or not, the longer other diseases like diabetes, high blood pressure and obesity are kept away.

Seasonal allergy sufferers, like my asthmatics, did notice a reduction in severity of symptoms. While most could not stop all their meds; the great majority were able to get better control of their allergic symptoms with fewer medications. For instance, if the allergy sufferer was taking three meds to control their allergies, they could get down to two or even one med with complete symptom control. This greatly improves a patient's ability to function on a daily basis, as they have to worry about taking less medication throughout the day.

RHEUMATOID ARTHRITIS

Rheumatoid arthritis (RA) is an autoimmune disease. Autoimmune means our bodies mistakenly believe certain parts of our own bodies are foreign, and then attack these body parts. In RA the part of the body being attacked are the joints. This can result in a debilitating disease where the person is unable to move the joints affected. Some people with RA become wheelchair bound, and some may become severely disabled in about ten years. Inflammation of the joints is what causes the severe debilitating aspect of this disease.

My first encounter with low carb diets and their possible relationship to RA, was in a book called *Neanderthin*, by Ray Audette. This book described the so-called 'cave man diet' and how it helped the author not only lose weight, hence the title, but also helped to alleviate his symptoms of RA. I would recommend this book to anyone who suffers from RA. I read this book after I was well into low carb diets and immediately saw the connection between low carbs, lessening of inflammation, and it's potential to help with the symptoms of RA.

I do suggest my RA sufferers begin low carb diets to help control pain. Unfortunately, our population is primed toward the use of pain meds, so I only have limited data on low carbs and RA. For those patients who began a very low carb regimen, that is, not more than twenty to twenty-four grams of carbs a day, definitive symptom improvement occurred. Some patients were able to reduce the amount of meds they needed to control their RA.

The other difficult aspect of RA is that most of my severe RA sufferers are elderly. The fact that they're elderly is not the difficult part; but try changing the diet of an octogenarian, well, I'm sure you get it. Most just look at me like I'm crazy and yes me to death. My younger RA sufferers are more amenable to changing their diets and the few that did were very thankful I told them about the RA-Carb connection.

EPILEPSY

Epilepsy occurs when nerve cells in the brain malfunction. If there is a large malfunction a grand mal seizure can result. This is the seizure where the person falls to the ground and shakes uncontrollably. Petit mal is another type of seizure commonly referred to as an absence seizure. This is the type of seizure where the person, usually a child, appears to be daydreaming. After a few seconds or maybe a minute the child returns to normal functioning.

My only knowledge of epilepsy and low carbs has been through the work of Dr. John Freeman. Dr. Freeman uses a ketogenic dietary approach in the treatment of severe epileptic children, who were not responding to typical drug therapy. He worked out of Johns Hopkins. There was a movie made depicting his success with his dietary approach in the treatment of severe epilepsy.

Ketogenic diets are similar to low carb diets in a sense that while they are comprised of low carbs, they also contain a high fat content. Even low carb diets are referred to as ketogenic, with ketogenic meaning 'ketone-producing.' This really is not a misnomer and I will sometimes refer to low carb diets as ketogenic, since the lower the carb intake, the more fat we use for fuel. Any diet that causes us to use fat for fuel will produce ketones, therefore, the term ketogenic could be used to describe the low carb diet I refer to in this book. The main difference is that the ketogenic diet Dr. Freeman uses contains more fat. The interesting thing that I found in his book was that they were concerned about the long-term effects of consuming high levels of fat. With an understanding of biochemistry this fear can be alleviated, as the consumption of more fat in the diet will not cause any new medical concerns. In fact, the more fat in the diet the less chance of seeing other things like diabetes, high blood pressure, or obesity, just to name a few.

The concern over children eating more fat comes from a priori reasoning, described in the first chapter of this book. It is the false belief that consuming a lot of fat is bad, but this is not true. The Eskimos have been doing it for thousands of years and they only have problems when they start eating more carbs. The bigger danger lies in the consumption of carbs, as has been explained throughout this book.

DEPRESSION

This is a disease I see quite often on a daily basis in my practice. I have told many of my depressed patients to lower their carbs and increase their fat, cholesterol and protein consumption. Most patients do feel better when they make this dietary change, and a few were able to stop their medications.

The most common medications used in the treatment of depression and anxiety are the selective serotonin re-uptake inhibitors. Even though we see the word inhibitor used to describe these meds, they actually *increase* the serotonin level in the blood. Interestingly enough, serotonin comes from the modification of the amino acid tryptophan. Amino acids come from the breakdown of proteins. Knowing this, I tell my depressed (or anxious) patients to increase their protein intake (by the way, turkey contains a lot of tryptophan), so their bodies will see more tryptophan, with conversion of the tryptophan, hopefully, into serotonin.

As an aside, what I haven't seen work to any substantial degree for depression are hypericin perforatum or s-adenosyl methionine. I have literally had hundreds of my patients try these products over the years and the patient's feedback, not mine, was these over the counter remedies did not work. Why do people buy these things? I suggest you read Michael Shermer's, *Why People Believe Weird Things,* for insight I cannot provide on these few pages.

DENTAL CARIES (TOOTH DECAY)

This should be a no-brainer. Eat too much sugar and your teeth develop cavities. The interesting thing is, when I suggest we should back off on carbs to lower our risk of dental caries, I get weird looks. The reason backing off on carbs will have a beneficial effect on our teeth, is because the less carbs we eat, the less sugar our teeth will see; the less sugar our teeth see, the less tooth decay will occur. It really is that simple.

I guess people think that it is the simple sugar, like what's in a candy bar that causes the problems with tooth decay. Trouble is, carbohydrates are broken down into simple sugars, and this process begins in our mouth, thanks to salivary amylase. These simple sugars then bathe the teeth and accelerate tooth decay. By lowering one's carb intake the teeth will be exposed to less sugar and we will have fewer problems with our teeth.

SLEEP APNEA (OBSTRUCTIVE)

Sleep apnea is a serious condition. It occurs when the smooth muscles of the neck relax too much, while we are sleeping, and inhibit our ability to breathe. Apnea literally means without breath. The current treatment is either to go to sleep with an apparatus known as a CPAP machine (which stands for Continuous Positive Airway Pressure), which delivers oxygen at high pressure, literally forcing the airways open; or to have an invasive surgery known as an uvulopalatopharyngoplasty (or UP3), where the ENT doc goes in and cuts away all the extra tissue.

If sleep apnea is not treated a myriad of medical problems can surface. Among these are high blood pressure, cardio-myopathy (an enlargement of the heart, which can lead to heart failure), muscle cramps, memory problems, light-headedness, and a condition known as narcolepsy, just to name a few. Narcolepsy is where a person falls asleep in seconds, as soon as they sit down, or attempt to drive a car. If one is driving a car and they fall asleep, well, I don't need to tell you the rest.

Most cases of sleep apnea are the obstructive sleep apnea type, which is seen in persons who are overweight. Sleep apnea can be cured by losing weight and we already know how to do this; by lowering our carb intake. I have seen patients stop using their CPAP machines after starting low carbs and losing weight. This is a common occurrence in my office. So, if you suffer from sleep apnea, low carbs is the way to go.

PAIN

We need substances called prostaglandins to feel pain. Prostaglandins come from arachidonate, which should be a household word for you by now. The more arachidonate in the body, the more pain.

Remember the path to arachidonate?

That's right;

it started with carbs;

which released insulin;

which created more arichidonate,

which created the prostaglandins,

which increased the pain.

By avoiding carbs we make less of the very things needed for us to feel pain. I have used the low carb approach to lower the pain experienced in patients with osteoarthritis, rheumatoid arthritis, IBD, colitis, chronic lower back pain (so long as they were not malingering, and you know who you are), in addition to any chronic pain producing illness and have seen remarkable reductions in pain, without the need for more meds.

If you are experiencing pain on a daily basis or even a few times a week, lower your carbs and monitor the effect. You should be lowering your carbs anyway because of the myriad of positive health benefits you will experience. Remember my cautionary advice in the prior chapters, if you are on meds for diabetes, blood pressure, or any other meds that you take on a daily basis, check with your doc before starting any low carb diet. If your doc tells you that low carb diets are dangerous and you shouldn't start low carbs; do yourself a favor and find another doctor who is comfortable with low carb diets.

CARDIAC ELECTRICAL DISTURBANCES

I first started low carbs on my patients with cardiac electrical disturbances after I read through Dr. Robert Atkins books. As a cardiologist he had noticed that certain electrical disturbances diminished and/or disappeared with the initiation of low carb diets. These electrical abnormalities were classified as premature atrial and premature ventricular rhythms.

I, too, have noticed a positive benefit when starting low carbs on this patient population. It did not prevent the need for meds to help with the electrical control of the heart, but it did lower the amount of skipped beats the patients felt and the amount I saw when their hearts were monitored for twenty-four hours. So, something good is happening. Sorry, I do not have a clue as to why these heart rhythms get better with low carbs, no one does. If these rhythms are due to inflammation, I can explain that, but I really do not have any idea why these abnormal heart rhythms get better. But they do, and I'm OK with that.

CHAPTER TWENTY-FIVE-CANCER

I was saving the worst for last. I did this on purpose because what we read last we tend to remember the best. If you remember anything from this book I want everyone to remember that I am convinced, both biochemically and clinically, that carbohydrates not only encourage the growth of new cancer cells, but allow cancer to spread once it has developed.

Our treatments for most types of cancer have progressed, but not to the point where we have effective cures. I know this statement will generate a lot of criticism especially from researchers in the cancer fields, but when it comes to most types of cancer, we really do not have effective cures. Yes, what we can offer medically is better than no care at all, but we really have not come across a super magic pill to cure all types of cancer. This would mean we would have to develop as many pills as there are cancers. And we never will.

This may seem like a pretty big thing to say. Some of you may think I should have said, "We *probably* will never develop a pill to cure each type of cancer." My reasoning behind why a pill to cure each type of cancer will never be developed is simple. Once cancer starts it is difficult, and for many cancers, impossible to stop. The best cure, and no one will disagree with me on this one, is prevention. Prevention of all types of cancer; but how can this be done?

The current thinking is that if we eat whole grains and a whole bunch of fruits and vegetables, we will be well on our way to preventing cancer. Oh yeah, avoid red meat too, and if you're going to eat any type of meat, make sure it's chicken and fish. Only problem is, this does not and has not worked to prevent cancer.

From this book you have learned that eating whole grains and fruits cause our cholesterols to go higher, we gain weight, our blood pressures elevate, and if we are unfortunate enough to carry the genes to be diabetic, our blood sugars will increase too.

So, the story goes, eat whole grains and fruits and you will prevent cancer. The only problem is that eating whole grains and fruits has not lowered the prevalence of cancers. For any of you who disagree with me, and I know there are a lot of you, just check and see how much cancer is still being diagnosed. Doctors are diagnosing new cases of cancer at an alarming rate, and I'm not talking about cancers related to smoking or exposure to chemicals known to cause cancer. I'm talking about the cancers where everyone, including the doctor, cannot figure out how or why the patient developed it in the first place. The most common types of cancers that fall into this category are the leukemias, multiple myelomas, colon cancers (in non smokers or drinkers), testicular, ovarian, brain, and any cancer where a reason for the cancer's development is a mystery.

It is very interesting that persons who are overweight, or even mildly overweight, tend to have higher cancer rates. We see this all the time as physicians. What doctor out there can provide you with the connection between being overweight and cancer?

I can.

It's insulin.

Insulin is the connection.

Why insulin? From the information contained in this book, we can now go through the biochemical pathway. It's easy, but we'll review it again.

People become overweight because of insulin. Remember, insulin is an anabolic hormone, it makes us bigger. I know there' s a lot of research on other things that may control weight gain, but these generally fall into the category of either appetite suppressants or appetite enhancers. The bottom line is if we eat carbs, we release insulin, and it is insulin that puts the weight on us. It's that simple. We spoke about this in the obesity chapter.

Now what happens biochemically when insulin is secreted? That's right, it travels to the cells of our body and in order for the cells to do what insulin wants, we need to use that second messenger system. This is where arachidonate was released, and in the body's attempt to get rid off arachidonate; we actually make the things which encourage cancer cells to grow and to spread. So, insulin's release will cause both a weight gain and encouragement of cancer cell growth. This is why persons who are heavier tend to get cancers more often.

I know doctors who are reading this will say they have patients who were quite skinny who developed cancers, who didn't smoke or drink; so what's up with that? They will think this disproves my theory on insulin as the starting point for the development of cancer.

It does not.

What I am saying is that insulin's presence allows the production of chemical mediators which have been widely implicated in cancer's start and spread. Our genetic disposition will tell our bodies what to do when exposed to higher levels of insulin. The problem is, just about everyone is exposed to higher levels of insulin, because most people are eating too many carbs.

If your genetic disposition is to gain weight if high levels of insulin are floating around in your blood, then you will gain weight. If heart disease is in your genes if your insulin level is elevated, then you get heart disease. If cancer is in your genes, then it's cancer. Our genes really control what our bodies do when exposed to higher levels of insulin.

Of course the patient who develops cancer needs to have the genes which cause cancer. These genes get the signal to turn on and start creating cancer cells from the breakdown products of arachidonate. Arachidonate's presence is influenced by insulin. The more insulin, the more arachidonate. The more arachidonate, the more signals get sent to cancer causing genes to start cancer growth. It is, unfortunately, that simple.

There is currently research being done which has implicated insulin-like molecules as a stimulus for breast cancer cell growth. Go to http://www.cancer.umn.edu/research/profiles/yee.html and review the web page. It's more startling once you know there is a connection between insulin and cancer. That web site only deals with breast cancer. We will find out over time that most, if not all, cancer growth is influenced by the presence of insulin.

This is scary stuff because most doctors do not know to

tell their patients to lower their carbs to lower their cancer risk, but will give all other useful tips as to how to prevent cancer. The biggest tip to lower cancer risk is not known by most doctors. Actually, I don't think any doctor I've spoken to even knows of the link between cancer and carbs.

Now here is something that's even more frightening, if that's possible. It is well known that cancer cells need to use sugar for a fuel source, without sugar, cancer cells die. I came across an article in a veterinary magazine years ago (I cannot find the article now, but I know it's out there) about using low carb diets to 'starve' cancer cells. It makes sense biochemically because if the cancer cells cannot get sugar, they will die. It gets a little complicated because cancer cells will take up the sugar in our blood and this will force the body to make more sugar. The question I have is this; if someone develops cancer, would a low carb, more fat, more cholesterol, more protein diet help kill off cancer cells? Could that be our best chemotherapeutic agent? We'd be hard pressed to find any studies of humans using this dietary approach because the researchers feel fat in the diet causes cancer. Does it? Sure, partially hydrogenated oils can and probably do, but what about the other, natural fats. I know more studies need to be performed where cancer patients are placed on low carb diets, along with more fat, more cholesterol and more protein, and then followed to see if there are any benefits. I know there will be benefits of doing this; I just hope the research starts soon.

So the bottom line is if you want to significantly lower your chances of developing any cancer, lower your carb intake and begin to eat more fat, cholesterol and protein. To those doctors who say eating fat causes or increases your cancer risk; let me see those studies and I will tell you how the study is flawed. As I've said earlier, any study which thinks it proves low carbs are dangerous, or that eating natural fat (and I include saturated fat in there too) is dangerous; I will show you how that study was performed improperly and really does not prove anything. It usually takes me less than a minute to point out the flaws in the study.

The diet studies out there, and there are probably thousands; rely on statistical interpretations to come to conclu-

sions. The problem with statistics, to quote Mark Twain, is

that "There are liars, there are damn liars, and then there's

statistics." Most of the researchers out there already know

the results they want and if the data do not support what

they feel should be the result, the data gets fudged; or the

results are reported with a bias. This means the researchers

manipulate either the data, or their interpretation of the

results, so it fits the conclusion they wanted.

For example, if a study shows that eating saturated fat low-

ers your risk of breast cancer, this would never get pub-

lished in any medical journal because all the doctors and

researchers have already made up their mind that this can't

be true. I picked breast cancer because there was a study

performed to attempt to prove that eating more fiber low-

ers your rate of colon cancer. The women participants

were divided up into five groups, where the first group ate

the least fiber and the fifth group ate the most fiber, with

the groups in between eating increasing amounts of fiber.

This study was supposed to prove what doctors already

thought they knew; that eating more fiber lowers your risk of colon cancer.

The problem was that when the data was analyzed, all five groups had the same amount of colon cancer. Oopps. This was a shocker, but who reading this knows about this study. It was never widely published because it went directly against what doctors thought they already knew. Quite frankly, even the researchers didn't understand the results.

We didn't understand the results because we had already made up our minds, without any proof, that eating fiber *has* to be good for us; this study suggested otherwise. So, instead of trying to figure out what the results really meant, the study's results just vanished.

A fascinating side note of the same study was that the women who ate the *most* saturated fat, had the *lowest* rates of breast cancer. That's right, the lowest rates, not the highest rates, as most doctors would suspect. Who remembers reading that in your daily paper, or seeing it on the evening news. Anyone? Again, instead of trying to figure out why these results occurred, this study just disappeared as well. Just for the record, this was a study with about 80,000 women, and that's a lot of women. The more persons in any statistical study, the more reliable the results depending on the way the study was set up, of course.

I want to take a few minutes to explain something about what doctors do clinically and why we do it. It may shock a lot of people reading this that for what us doctors do clinically, there may not have been any studies performed to prove what we are doing is even the right thing to do. As I mentioned in the beginning of this book, when we go to medical school and throughout our internships, residencies and even after we graduate; we treat our patients as we were told to treat them. Unfortunately, there may be very few studies done to support what we are told to do and how we are instructed to treat our patients. This is especially true when it comes to dietary advice.

Does this scare anyone?

It should.

It scared me after I figured it out. Ignorance really is bliss. Thank goodness we now have something called evidenced based medicine. Evidenced based medicine is where studies are actually performed to see if what us doctors are doing clinically, really adds any benefit to patient outcomes. Any doctor whose read through these wonderful books (and I'm not being sarcastic, I really think they're wonderful) is usually shocked. As an example, all us doctors who treat newborns think we know that mylicon works to get rid of a newborn's gas. Parents swear by it. But when this treatment was actually studied, the study showed no clinical benefit between using mylicon versus not using anything. This certainly shocked me.

It's nice to know that the medical profession is finally studying clinical outcomes, so doctors treating you can actually point to a study to prove what we're doing is more effective than not doing anything at all. Only problem is, I'm still waiting for the low carb, more fat, more cholesterol, and more protein studies.

How long will I have to wait?

I'm going to change gears a little bit and take a look at how much my medical profession's ignorance costs us on a yearly basis. I wrote a research paper during my MBA studies which focused on that very topic. The results were astounding.

The final chapter of my story will attempt to examine why physicians believe low fat, low cholesterol diets work. I am grateful to Michael Shermer's book, *Why People Believe Weird Things?* This book stimulated my curiosity as to why intelligent people, that is, doctors, would believe in and continue to suggest something that just doesn't work.

CHAPTER TWENTY-SIX-THE ECONOMIC
IMPLICATIONS OF PHYSICIAN'S
DIETARY IGNORANCE.

Throughout this book I have been wearing my medical hat.
Now it's time for me to put on my business hat.

Most people with insurance who are not on any medications do not care much about economic implications, as
they believe their insurance absorbs the costs of whatever
disease they may come down with. Unless, of course, you
are someone with coronary artery disease or diabetes. If
you are, then you know that many times when your doctor
attempts to give you a medication, your insurance company wants you on a different medication, what the insurance company euphemistically refers to as a 'preferred'
agent.

What preferred means, and all that it means, is that your insurance company has a financial agreement with a particular

pharmaceutical company, to use only their product for a particular disease. This way the pharmaceutical company can drop the cost a little, because they will make up any lost profit by selling more products. Do not think that 'preferred' means it is better for you, because sometimes the preferred medication may not be as effective. Only your doctor can tell you if a preferred medication is as safe and effective as the other medication you were taking.

Whenever a pharmacist dispenses a medication, someone is paying for that medication. Even if your plan's co-pay for a particular medication is only two dollars; if the medication costs fifty dollars to someone without insurance, the forty-eight dollars to make up the difference has to come from somewhere.

Where does that money come from? Well, it generally comes from the monthly insurance premiums you pay, or, as above, from agreements made between pharmaceutical and insurance companies to keep prices lower. But the bottom line is that someone, somewhere, eventually has to pay for that medication.

Trouble is, the newer the medication, the higher the cost. Newer medications do not necessarily mean better, but patients think so, and pharmaceutical companies market the newer medications as being better than the older ones. Patients are now presenting to our offices asking, oftentimes demanding, these newer products. Remember, these newer medications cost more. Even though the patient may not pay the entire cost for the medication, as mentioned above, somebody, somewhere, eventually pays for the medication.

Who do you think pays for the newer, more expensive products? You do; in the form of higher co-pays and higher monthly premiums. Don't think you're off the hook if your company pays for your insurance, because if your company is paying higher premiums, you lose out somehow. The way employees usually lose out is that the higher monthly insurance premiums prevent us employers from getting involved in 401k plans, or retirement plans for our employees. Or it could translate into a lower or no yearly bonus. Or employers are forced into having their employees pay a percentage of their health care costs. Suffice it to say that the higher the monthly insurance premium, the more everyone loses.

The above is important to point out, as this chapter deals with how doctor's dietary ignorance affects health care costs, and how the plain and simple act of lowering one's carbs can save these costs. I was going to research the cost savings for all the diseases mentioned in part two of my book, but I only had to research three. The reason I stopped at three is because the cost savings was so large it shocked me, and I was afraid to proceed any further. Suffice it to say I do like occasional ignorant bliss. The three diseases I researched were coronary artery disease (CAD), Type II diabetes mellitus (Type II DM), and gastro-esophageal reflux disease (GERD). I wanted to examine the costs associated with CAD, as it is the number one killer of both female and male Americans. If we could get all Americans to lower their carbs, and eat more protein, fat and cholesterol, the CAD rates, and most other disease processes, would drop to near zero.

I know there will be a large amount of skepticism with this comment, but that's ok. I prefer skepticism to cynicism, as skeptics tend to want to disprove a statement by running experiments and analyzing data, while cynics just sit back and let their opinions take precedence. Cynics do nothing to help prove or disprove, they are antithetical to progress. A cynic will not perform any experiment to try to prove or disprove anything, as they are already thoroughly convinced their way is the right way. Unfortunately, you will find most of your cynics in the medical profession. And this will not help disseminate proper dietary information. Now let's get back to some numbers. Using data from 2002 there was approximately 65.7 billion dollars spent on coronary artery bypass grafts and angioplasties alone. Go to http://www.brookings.edu/comm./policybriefs/ pb148.pdf. It is important to note that not included in this figure is the amount spent on medications by patients each year that had these procedures done. Where do you think the 65.7 billion is coming from? That's right, somehow, somewhere, it's coming out of *your* pocket.

Moving on to Type II diabetes, it cost 22.9 billion dollars a year to treat a Type II diabetic. As a particular web site stated," 22.9 billion dollars a year was three times the cost for medical care than a patient without diabetes." The director of this particular research project, which derived this number stated, "It really points out the importance of managing the disease." Lowering the carbs, and eating more cholesterol, more fat and more protein would lower the costs associated with Type II DM virtually to zero. I wonder how the director of the study would respond to that.

So with CAD and Type II DM, if we lower the carb intake, and eat more protein, fat and cholesterol, we would save 88.6 **billion** dollars a year.

That's 88.6 **billion** dollars a year!

And remember for CAD I used 2002 figures, not 2007 as these were not available, which means the CAD costs will be even higher. Based on the figures I'm using for CAD and Type II DM that's nearly a **hundred billion** dollars!

A hundred billion dollars saved just by lowering one's carb intake!

When are *we* going to wake up?! By 'we' I mean us doctors, the insurance companies and yes, our government as well.

Don't think for even a second your insurance company is not familiar with these cost figures, they are. It is your insurance company's primary objective to keep the costs associated with CAD and Type II DM as low as possible. They keep these costs down; they get to keep more money. What's better than that? So why is it that even the insurance companies are not promoting the importance of low carb dieting? The insurance companies are not promoting the importance of low carb diets because they generally adhere to the mainstream *accepted* dietary regimens. They believe in the a priori approach and it costs them almost a hundred billion a year. Oh well, is that the price to pay for poetic justice? Remember, it's you who are paying the costs associated with your insurance company's dietary ignorance. The insurance companies just get to keep less of your money because of their ignorance, but it's still *your* money.

Putting on my legal hat, they are probably aware of the studies performed which support low carb dieting, but are still afraid of the low carb diet because it entails eating more fat and more cholesterol. The insurance companies most likely fear litigation from their customers (that's you by the way, if you have insurance), as they are uncertain if eating more fat and more cholesterol is dangerous or not. This is not necessarily a bad thing, that is, to be uncertain of the outcomes of eating more fat and more cholesterol; but I know I am not the only doctor out there using low carbs as a tool to help keep my patients healthier and disease free.

As an interesting side note, I remember one of the insurance companies I accept wanted me to disseminate incorrect dietary information to my diabetic patients. I politely refused, simply stating that I prefer to give my patients my own dietary information. It wasn't soon after that I was told I was being audited, specifically my diabetic patient's charts were being requested for review by the insurance company. After the audit, the examiners could not believe how well controlled my diabetic patients were. They used the HgBA1c and microalbuminuria as criteria of control, among others.

My point of all this is that the insurance companies are so sure they are using the correct dietary guidelines, they want to instill these guidelines into every practice in America. If the insurance companies knew they could save up to, and probably more, than a hundred billion a year with low carb diets, they'd be forcing their customers to follow a low carb diet. So I guess I should be happy that the dietary ignorance killing all of us does not fall on the shoulders of doctors alone. Yes, your insurance company is part of the problem too, as they have not learned how to think for themselves dietarily yet. Will it ever happen? Only time will tell. Since insurance companies are motivated by profit, I say it will happen sooner rather than later, as far as the insurance companies are concerned.

But hold on, there's more. I also researched some cost figures on gastro-esophageal reflux disease (GERD); another disease effectively treated and oftentimes eliminated with low carb diets. The costs here were so utterly staggering I almost fell down. In 2005 figures America lost 2 **BILLION** dollars a **WEEK** on diminished productivity in the workplace, due to the symptoms associated with GERD. That's 2 BILLION dollars a WEEK!!!! Calculating it out, that's 104 BILLION dollars a year.

So let's add it all up. Between CAD, Type II DM and GERD, Americans spent over **ONE HUNDRED NINETY TWO BILLION DOLLARS** on just three diseases alone. Yes, that money could have been saved if people followed a low carb, more fat, more cholesterol, and more protein diet. Remember, every one of us is paying the price for eating too many carbs, and not enough protein, fat and cholesterol.

CHAPTER TWENTY-SEVEN-WHY DO DOCTOR'S BELIEVE LOW FAT, LOW CHOLESTEROL DIETS WORK?

It has been over nine years since I started using low carb diets in my practice. I started myself on a low carb diet first, before I implemented low carb diets into my practice. After I saw the wonderful benefits on myself, that is, the weight loss, the raising of my HDL, the lowering of my blood pressure; I wanted to start more of my patients on low carb diets.

I guess I was still a bit apprehensive, so before I started low carbs on my patients, I got my family and friends to try it out to see how they did. I was still in the early stages of learning about low carb diets, and even though I understood the biochemistry behind why low carb diets were safe and effective, I was still uncertain if low carbs would be the right thing for everyone. We have all seen cases where a particular diet works great for one person, but when others try it, it either doesn't work or bad things happen. And I figured if I was wrong and bad stuff happened to my family and friends, I had a low chance of being sued. Also, I was the only person I had tried the diet on, and so I naturally wondered if it would work on others.

The result of starting my family and friends on a low carb, more protein, fat and cholesterol diet was that they all did great. They lost weight, blood pressures dropped, lipid profiles changed dramatically for the better, and those with diabetes realized better control of their blood sugars. Everyone who started low carbs and I mean everyone, realized a significant benefit, and, no, I didn't get sued.

So then I decided to begin low carb diets in my practice. Cautiously at first and with strict follow-ups, usually on a weekly basis, coupled with daily phone calls. The first few patients I started on low carbs did great. After the first trial, and after I saw the benefits incurred by my patients, I began low carbs on just about anyone who was willing to try it. They all did fantastic. For the first time in my clinical career I was able to stop medications, get better control over blood sugars, and patients who I had a difficult time controlling blood pressures or blood sugars, became more easily manageable.

It wasn't soon after I began implementing low carbs into my patient's lives that I became angry that I had given thousands of patients the wrong dietary information. The wrong dietary information I am referring to is the low fat, low cholesterol diet, which I had instructed patients to follow when I was a medical student, intern and resident, and for at least five years as a physician in private practice. I argued with myself, to make myself feel better of course, that I had not done it on purpose; I was only following the accepted guidelines. It did nothing to console me that I had still given thousands, more likely tens of thousands of patients, the wrong dietary information over the years. I had had an active role in worsening people's medical problems and I felt miserable about it. I couldn't sleep for months. My anger at my profession for their continued ignorance and downright refusal to accept the positive benefits of low carb diets, changed to frustration and then into bewilderment. I am presently at a stage where since I have seen thousands upon thousands of my patients benefit from a low carb diet, that I now approach my profession in regards to diet, like I would approach a kindergarten student who thinks one plus one equals three. Why bother argue, you are not going to change the kindergarten's belief that one and one is not three, just like you will not change the belief of the doctor who still holds on tenaciously to the idea that low fat, low cholesterol diets are safe.

Notice what word I am using to describe how the kindergarten child or the doctor maintains their position. I am using the word *belief.* Sometimes beliefs turn out to be true, sometimes not. Some of us used to believe in Santa Claus, the Easter Bunny, or the tooth fairy, but we now know these are not real characters. (I did not know if I should capitalize bunny or not, so I took the safe way out, out of respect for the Easter Bunny of course.)

It is difficult to change someone's belief. Try changing one's political or religious beliefs. We all know this is virtually impossible and if we have a modicum of intelligence, we'll stay far away from these topics in ordinary conversation. The same is true with our dietary beliefs. I have found out over the last nine years that some people hold on to the belief that low fat, low cholesterol diets are the way to go, and will not change this thinking no matter what evidence I present to them. Oftentimes, it is the most stubborn of my patients, who, when they finally start following low carbs and realize the benefits, become my most loyal supporters of the low carb diet.

A great example of this was when I had the privilege to care for an extremely insightful and intelligent RN who thought I was absolutely crazy for wanting to increase her fat and cholesterol consumption. She knew all too well what the current dietary recommendations were, as she would counsel her own patients dietarily on a daily basis. So I approached my conversation with her in a very logical and instructive format, explaining biochemically what happens when one eats fat, cholesterol, carbs and protein. She listened attentively to every detail as I explained it to her. At the end of the discussion she raised an eyebrow and commented, "So you mean to tell me, I can continue to have my egg mcmuffin in the morning, taking the top muffin off, eat even more cholesterol and fat, lower my carbs, and my cholesterol profile will improve and I'll lose weight."

I responded in the affirmative.

Three months later when I revealed her lab tests to her, she was amazed. She already suspected her numbers would be better, as she had lost weight; but she was absolutely astounded to see her HDL had increased, despite the fact she knew she was eating more cholesterol. She immediately became angry with the medical profession for their continued ignorance of low carb diets, and I confided in her I had felt the same emotions.

I stated to her that I did not think the medical profession was acting malevolently, that it was just being cautious as to not jump into things too quickly, before all the studies were in. But she then asked me why did *I* know about low carbs and why was *I* using low carbs in my practice before all the studies were in. I did not have an answer for her. I could only help but wonder, "Why *do* most docs continue to believe in low fat, low cholesterol diets?" It was not until I read Michael Shermer's, *Why People Believe Weird Things*, that I finally had my answer. Of course, 'people' would refer to doctors here, and the 'weird thing' would be doctors believing a low fat, low cholesterol diet works.

So why do doctors believe low fat, low cholesterol diets are safe and effective when they are not. It's quite simple. I already explained that in medical school and residency we are not taught to be free thinkers, we are taught what the faculty thinks we need to know, and we are told, either implicitly or explicitly, not to question what we are being told. In chapter eighteen of Why *People Believe Weird Things*, Michael Shermer makes the comment "Students are taught what to think, not how to think." I could not agree more with Dr. Shermer. It is the way we students are taught that prohibits (inhibits?) most of us from breaking out of our shells and thinking for ourselves.

As an aside, I remember being in pharmacy class in medical school when the instructor was talking about statins.

Statins are the most popular drugs used to lower cholesterol. The instructor made a comment that these drugs can lower one's heart attack risk by up to thirty-five percent. I then asked, "Do you mean that out of *all* the people on these drugs, only *thirty-five percent* experienced a reduction in heart disease?"

The instructor responded, "That is correct." Obviously not noticing, or ignoring, my sarcasm.

I then asked, " So this means that *sixty-five percent* of the people taking these medications are still having heart attacks?"

The instructor got annoyed with this comment and stated, "Yes, well, why that may be true, this is the best we have to offer."

The best we have to offer? Am I the only one who gets it? I know I'm not. I should have figured it all out then, but I remained ignorant for many years to follow.

When we are told low fat, low cholesterol diets are safe and effective from the get go, that is, starting in first grade all the way through college and residency; when we continue to be bombarded with this same notion, again and again and again; when all we know is low fat, low cholesterol; we assimilate this as a belief, and we do not question its veracity. Unless, of course, we stop and think for ourselves.

The reason patients continue to be placed on low fat, low cholesterol diets is because doctors actually believe these diets are safe and effective. They really, truly, honestly believe in their heart of hearts, that low fat, low cholesterol dieting is the way to go. When someone believes that strongly in something, there is no way they are going to change their minds, even if the evidence is overwhelming. On top of that, doctors will use language that appears intelligent and logical to defend the position that low fat, low cholesterol diets are safe and effective.

Chapter eighteen of Dr. Shermer's *Why People Believe Weird Things* is titled, Why Do Smart People Believe Weird Things. Dr. Shermer's answer as to why smart people believe weird things is, "Smart people believe weird things because they are skilled at defending beliefs they arrived at for non-smart reasons." When I read that sentence I almost shouted out Eureka! To me it made perfect sense. I remembered when I was being told by friends and patients about low carbs before I knew the truth; about how wonderful they felt on low carbs; about how much weight they were losing; and about how those with medical conditions were able to stop some of their medications. I recall like it was yesterday coming up with a myriad of reasons why they should not follow a low carb diet.

I would shout out things like hepatic steatosis, proteinuria, medial monckenberg's sclerosis, hypertension, and the like. Yes, I would use those words and of course nobody knew what I was talking about. Not even myself. But the words sounded pretty scary and most people would be frightened enough to stop the low carb diet.

Man was I stupid. Or was I? Could it be that I was just defending a belief system that had been indoctrinated into me over the years? A belief system so ingrained in me that I would defend it no matter what, even if what I was saying were untrue? I certainly was good defending my belief, and yes, all it was, was the belief, that low fat, low cholesterol diets are safer than low carb diets. I definitely had the skills to defend a position I arrived at for 'non-smart reasons.' I am utterly embarrassed to say I had dissuaded thousands of people from starting a low carb diet, simply because I was skillful at defending my incorrect position that low carb diets were dangerous. Thank goodness I woke up, but of course I'm forever frightened and wonder about what other things I am ignorant about. I wish I could say ignorance is bliss, but I cannot. I cannot because due to the medical profession's continued dietary ignorance, millions of people are dying each year, and as long as this dietary ignorance persists, millions of people will continue to die each and every year. Yes, it is we doctors who are causing millions to die, and, yes, this does constitute GENO-CIDE!!!!

Well I guess this brings me to the end of my story for now. Thanks for letting me share with you what I have learned over the last nine years. I'm glad you took the time to read what I had to say. I'm sure there will be fallout on my side; there usually is when the truth is told. I only hope that everyone and I mean everyone throughout the world, are made aware of the dangers inherent in carbohydrates, and avoid, like the plague, low fat, and low cholesterol diets.

HIGHLY SUGGESTED READINGS;

Protein Power and Protein Power Life Plan, Eades & Eades MD, any edition.

New Diet Revolution, Robert Atkins MD, any edition.

Neanderthin, Ray Audette

The Zone, Barry Sears PhD

The Ketogenic Diet, John Freeman MD (A book specifically for those who treat epilepsy)

3193635

Made in the USA